The Methane SIBO & IMO Handbook

Intestinal Methanogen Overgrowth and Why It Needs a Different Approach When Bloating and Stubborn Constipation Won't Budge.

Allegria Mackenzie Giraffe

First Edition

ISBN: 979-8-90599-296-4

Medical Disclaimer

This book is for education and general information only. It is not medical advice, and it is not a substitute for diagnosis or treatment by a qualified clinician who knows your history. The conditions discussed here, including intestinal methanogen overgrowth, are diagnosed and treated by physicians and other licensed professionals. Nothing in these pages should be read as a recommendation to start, stop, combine, or dose any medication, antibiotic, herbal antimicrobial, or supplement on your own. Antibiotics in particular are prescription medicines with real risks, and the treatment combinations described are presented so that you can understand them and discuss them with a prescriber, never so that you can attempt them without one. The author is writing under a pen name and is not your clinician. If you have symptoms that concern you, or if your symptoms change suddenly, contact a medical professional. Names and identifying details in every case example have been changed or are composites, and no example describes a real, identifiable person.

Table of Contents

Preface

You have probably been told, more than once, that what you have is irritable bowel syndrome. Maybe you were told it kindly, maybe briskly, maybe by someone who had already stood up to open the door. Either way, you left with a label that explained nothing and a suggestion to eat more fiber, drink more water, and manage your stress. You tried. The bloating still arrived every afternoon like a scheduled appointment. The constipation still refused to answer to anything you threw at it. And somewhere along the way you found the word SIBO, and then you found that your version of it came with an asterisk, because people kept telling you that yours was the difficult kind.

They were half right. Your overgrowth may indeed be the kind that behaves differently, resists the standard playbook, and comes back after treatment that should have worked. What almost nobody explained is why. That why is the whole subject of this book.

The short version is that the organisms driving your symptoms are probably not bacteria at all. They are archaea, a separate branch of life, and they make methane, and methane does something specific to your gut that hydrogen does not. That single fact reorganizes everything: why you are constipated rather than loose, why one round of the usual antibiotic underperformed, why your treatment keeps unraveling a few months later. The field has a newer name for this picture, intestinal methanogen overgrowth, or IMO, and the name is not a rebranding exercise. It is a correction, and the correction points directly at what actually helps.

I have written this as a serious book for an intelligent reader who is tired of being handed pamphlets. It does not promise a cure, because the honest evidence does not support that promise. It grades what is known, flags what is shaky, and refuses to oversell. What it will do is give you a clear, mechanistic understanding of your own gut and a set of specific, informed questions to bring to the clinician who can actually help you. That combination, understanding plus leverage, is worth more than one more list of foods to avoid.

Read it in order if you can. Each chapter is built on the one before it, and the argument accumulates.

Introduction

The sentence that sends most people to a book like this one is some version of "your SIBO is just harder to treat." It is a strange thing to be told. It names a problem and withholds the reason in the same breath. You are left knowing only that you are on the wrong side of some line, without being told where the line is or how you ended up there.

This book is written to draw that line clearly. The reason your case behaves differently is not that you are unlucky or noncompliant or somehow more broken than the next patient. It is that the microorganism at the center of your symptoms belongs to a different domain of life, follows different rules, and produces a different gas, and that gas changes how your entire digestive tract moves. Once you see that, the rest stops being mysterious. The constipation makes sense. The treatment failures make sense. The relapses make sense.

A brief word on what this book is and is not. It is an explanatory handbook. It teaches you the biology, the diagnosis, the treatment logic, and the maintenance strategy in enough depth that you can hold your own in a specialist's office. It is not a protocol you administer to yourself. The most effective treatments discussed in these pages involve prescription antibiotics used in specific combinations, and those decisions belong to a prescriber who has examined you. When the text explains why two antibiotics beat one, it is arming you for a conversation, not handing you a regimen. Hold that distinction firmly, because it is the difference between a well-informed patient and a person who got hurt trying to shortcut the system.

You will also notice that this book is careful about evidence. Some of what is known about intestinal methanogen overgrowth rests on strong physiology and repeated observation. Some rests on small studies, retrospective chart reviews, and expert consensus that the experts themselves rate as low quality. I tell you which is which. That honesty is not hedging. It is the single thing that separates a trustworthy guide from the confident content that has probably already wasted your money.

Here is the path the book takes. Chapter 1 establishes what you are actually dealing with: archaea, not bacteria, and why the name IMO is more accurate than the name SIBO. Chapter 2 teaches you to read your own breath test without panic. Chapter 3 explains the mechanism that defines your subtype, the way methane slows your gut. Chapter 4 resolves the daily frustration of constipation that fiber and laxatives never fix. Chapter 5 explains why the standard treatment underperformed for you specifically. Chapter 6 walks through the combined antimicrobial approach in patient terms. Chapter 7 gives herbal options a fair, evidence graded hearing. Chapter 8 makes the case that motility, not just killing organisms, is the whole game. Chapter 9 builds an eating approach that lowers fermentation without starving your gut. Chapter 10 helps you hunt for the root cause so you can stop chasing symptoms. Chapter 11 prepares you for the doctor who says it is just IBS. And Chapter 12 addresses the part nobody puts in these books, the mental weight of living inside a body that has stopped cooperating.

Before you turn the page, do one small thing. Write down your three worst symptoms and, if you have a breath test result, the highest methane number on it. You will use both throughout this book, and the act of naming them precisely is the first step out of the fog.

Chapter 1.0: The Archaea Behind the Overgrowth

Here is a claim that sounds wrong the first time you hear it. The condition you have been calling bacterial overgrowth is very likely not bacterial. The organisms multiplying in your gut and generating the gas that makes your afternoons miserable are not bacteria in the ordinary sense at all. They belong to a separate domain of life, one that diverged from bacteria so long ago that the two are less like cousins and more like different kingdoms with a superficial resemblance. That single reclassification, from bacteria to archaea, is the key that unlocks everything else in this book, and it is why the field has quietly moved from calling your condition methane dominant SIBO to calling it intestinal methanogen overgrowth.

1.1 A Different Branch of Life

Biologists sort all living things into three great domains: bacteria, eukaryotes, and archaea. You and every plant, animal, and fungus are eukaryotes, organisms whose cells package their DNA inside a nucleus. Bacteria are the familiar single celled organisms that live nearly everywhere, cause many infections, and populate the healthy gut in enormous numbers. Archaea are the third branch, and they are the one almost no one learns about in school. They were only recognized as a separate domain in the late twentieth century, when genetic sequencing revealed that certain microbes long assumed to be unusual bacteria were in fact profoundly different at the molecular level.

The archaea that matter for your gut are the methanogens, so named because they make methane. The dominant one, present in the human digestive tract of most people at low levels, is a species called Methanobrevibacter smithii (Villanueva-Millan et al., 2022).

In a balanced gut it sits quietly at a small fraction of the total microbial population. When it overgrows, the fraction rises, methane output climbs, and symptoms follow.

Why does this taxonomic detail matter to a person who just wants to stop being bloated and constipated? Because the differences between archaea and bacteria are not academic. Archaea build their cell walls out of different materials than bacteria do. They run different metabolic machinery. And, critically for treatment, they do not respond to many of the antibiotics designed to kill bacteria, because those drugs target structures that archaea simply do not have. When a clinician reaches for the standard bacterial overgrowth prescription and your methane barely moves, this is why. The drug was built for a target you are not carrying in abundance.

1.2 Why the Old Name Misleads

The term SIBO stands for small intestinal bacterial overgrowth, and for the methane dominant patient every word of it is at least partly wrong. Consider the pieces. The overgrowth is not primarily bacterial, it is archaeal. And it is not confined to the small intestine either. When researchers measure methanogens in people with high breath methane, they find elevated levels in stool as well, which means the organisms are flourishing throughout the intestinal tract, colon included, not just in the small bowel where classic bacterial overgrowth occurs (Pimentel et al., 2020). Two of the three defining words in the old name do not describe your condition accurately.

This is why the American College of Gastroenterology and the authors of the North American Consensus moved toward the term intestinal methanogen overgrowth (Pimentel et al., 2020; Rezaie et al., 2017). The new name keeps only what is true. It says intestinal, not small intestinal, because the organisms range more widely. It says methanogen, naming the actual culprit, rather than bacterial.

And it says overgrowth, which remains accurate. The label change is a piece of intellectual honesty catching up with the biology.

None of this means the word SIBO is banished. You will still hear clinicians, testing companies, and other patients say methane SIBO or methane dominant SIBO, and you will know what they mean. The terms are used more or less interchangeably in conversation. But the reason IMO is worth adopting is that it carries the mechanism inside the name. Every time you say intestinal methanogen overgrowth, you are reminding yourself and everyone in the room that the target is an archaeon that makes methane, which is exactly the fact that determines what will and will not help you.

1.3 What Methanogens Actually Do

Methanogens make their living through a chemical trick. They consume hydrogen and carbon dioxide and combine them to produce methane. In your gut, the hydrogen comes largely from ordinary bacteria fermenting the carbohydrates you eat. Those bacteria release hydrogen as a waste product, and under normal conditions some of that hydrogen would build up. Methanogens step in and mop it up, using it as fuel and releasing methane in return.

This relationship is called cross feeding, and it explains a pattern you may have noticed on your own breath test. People with significant methanogen overgrowth often show low hydrogen and high methane, because the archaea are consuming the hydrogen almost as fast as the bacteria produce it and converting it to methane. If you went into your test expecting the diarrhea associated hydrogen picture and came out with a methane result instead, the cross feeding relationship is the reason the numbers looked upside down.

The methane these organisms produce is not an inert byproduct that simply leaves your body. It is biologically active inside the gut, and what it does to your intestinal muscle is the subject of Chapter 3. For now, hold onto the outline of the story. Bacteria ferment your food and make hydrogen. Archaea eat the hydrogen and make methane. The methane then acts on the muscular wall of your intestine in a way that slows everything down. That slowing is the origin of your constipation, and it also, in a cruel loop, makes the overgrowth easier to sustain. A slow gut does not clear itself efficiently, and organisms that would otherwise be swept along get to linger and multiply.

1.4 Common Misunderstandings

Several ideas about methane overgrowth circulate widely and are worth correcting before they mislead you.

The first is that methane overgrowth is simply a more severe version of ordinary SIBO, as if it sat further along the same scale. It does not. It is a different phenomenon driven by a different organism producing a different gas with a different effect on the bowel. Treating it as severe hydrogen SIBO, which is precisely what happens when a clinician applies the standard single antibiotic approach, is one of the most common reasons methane patients fail to improve.

The second misunderstanding is that a high methane number means you are severely ill, and a modest one means you are barely affected. The diagnostic threshold, a methane reading of ten parts per million or more at any point during a breath test, tells you that methanogens are overgrown, but the number does not map neatly onto how bad you will feel (Rezaie et al., 2017). Some people with numbers just over the threshold are miserable. Others with higher numbers are managing. Chapter 2 will help you interpret your own result in context rather than treating the figure as a verdict.

The third misunderstanding is that because these are not really bacteria, ordinary antibiotics are useless and you should skip straight to natural remedies. This is half true and dangerously oversimplified. Standard single antibiotics do underperform against archaea, which is real. But specific antibiotic combinations, discussed at length in Chapter 6, work considerably better than either the single drug approach or most of what is sold as a natural alternative. The lesson is not that medicine has nothing to offer. It is that the right medicine looks different for you than it does for the hydrogen dominant patient.

The following account is a composite, with details changed for anonymity.

Merritt had been through three rounds of the same nonabsorbable antibiotic over about a year, each prescribed for what her notes called SIBO. Each round bought her perhaps a month of easier mornings before the bloating and the straining crept back. By the third round she had concluded that she was one of those people for whom nothing works, and she had started reading forums late at night looking for someone with her exact story. What she eventually learned, from a gastroenterologist who actually looked at her breath test rather than her diagnosis code, was that her methane had never meaningfully dropped on any of those rounds. The drug she had taken three times was reasonable for a hydrogen dominant patient and close to the wrong tool for hers. The relief she had felt each time was partly the accompanying diet change and partly regression toward her own baseline, not the antibiotic clearing the archaea. Nothing about her was treatment resistant. She had simply been treated, three times, for a condition she did not have.

Merritt's story is not unusual, and it is not a story about a bad doctor. It is a story about a label, SIBO, that quietly instructs everyone to reach for the bacterial playbook even when the patient in front of them is carrying an archaeal problem. The name change to IMO exists precisely to interrupt that reflex.

1.5 Seeing the Difference in Practice

The clearest way to feel the weight of the archaea versus bacteria distinction is to watch how two similar looking patients diverge once the underlying organism is identified.

The following are composite cases.

Hollis arrived with months of bloating, loose stools, and urgency. His breath test showed a brisk early rise in hydrogen and negligible methane. He was treated as a hydrogen dominant patient, given a single nonabsorbable antibiotic for the standard course, and told to reduce fermentable carbohydrates for a few weeks. He responded well. His stools firmed up, the urgency eased, and while he needed attention to the reasons his gut had become hospitable to overgrowth in the first place, the initial treatment did roughly what it was supposed to do.

Tierney arrived with a story that sounded similar on the surface, bloating and abdominal discomfort that worsened through the day. But her dominant complaint was the opposite of Hollis's. She was constipated, often going days without a proper bowel movement, and her bloating felt trapped rather than gassy. Her breath test showed low hydrogen and methane well above the threshold. Given the same single antibiotic Hollis received, she barely improved. Only when a clinician recognized the methane picture and treated it as an archaeal problem, with the combined approach described later in this book and a serious plan for her sluggish motility, did she begin to see durable change.

The contrast is the entire point. Hollis and Tierney presented with overlapping symptoms and were separated by a single feature on a breath test, the gas their gut was producing. That one feature pointed to two different organisms, two different mechanisms, and two different treatment paths. When both patients are filed under the same three letter label, Tierney gets Hollis's treatment and quietly fails on it. When the methane picture is named for what it is, her path forward becomes visible.

1.6 What the Name Change Buys You

The reclassification from methane dominant SIBO to intestinal methanogen overgrowth is easy to dismiss as jargon, one more acronym in a field already crowded with them. That would be a mistake, because for you the new name is not a label, it is a set of instructions. It tells you that your overgrowth is archaeal, which tells you why single antibiotics disappoint. It tells you that methanogens make methane, which tells you why you are constipated rather than loose. It tells you the organisms range beyond the small intestine, which tells you why the problem can feel so diffuse and so stubborn.

Everything that follows in this book is, in a sense, an unfolding of the name. The chapters on treatment explain how to target an archaeon rather than a bacterium. The chapters on motility explain how to counter the slowing effect of methane. The chapters on diet explain how to reduce the hydrogen supply that feeds the whole cross feeding cycle. Hold the central fact steady as you read, that you are dealing with a methane making organism from a separate branch of life, and the rest of the book will read less like a collection of tips and more like a single argument that finally accounts for your experience.

Chapter 2.0: Reading Your Breath Test

You are holding a piece of paper, or looking at a PDF on your phone, and it is covered in numbers that mean nothing to you. There is a line for hydrogen and a line for methane, a column of time points running from zero to a hundred and twenty minutes, and somewhere a note saying positive or elevated that has done nothing to calm you down. Someone charged you real money for this, and then either handed it back without explanation or attached a one line interpretation that raised more questions than it answered. This chapter teaches you to read the thing yourself, so that the number on the page stops being a source of dread and starts being usable information.

2.1 What the Test Actually Measures

A breath test for intestinal methanogen overgrowth is built on a simple idea. You swallow a measured dose of a sugar the test uses as bait, and then over the next two to three hours you breathe into a collection device at set intervals. The sugar travels through your gut, and if organisms are present that ferment it, they release gases. Some of those gases cross from your intestine into your bloodstream, travel to your lungs, and leave in your breath, where the machine can measure them (Saad & Chey, 2014). The test is not measuring the organisms directly. It is measuring the gases they exhale on your behalf, which is why breath testing is a reasonable and noninvasive stand in for the far more invasive alternative of sampling fluid from the small intestine.

Two gases matter most. Hydrogen is produced by ordinary bacteria fermenting the sugar. Methane is produced by the archaea, the methanogens, that this book is about. A newer generation of tests also measures a third gas, hydrogen sulfide, but for your purposes the methane line is the one to find first. It is the line that tells you whether the organisms driving your constipation are overgrown (Rezaie et al., 2017).

The sugar used as bait is usually either glucose or lactulose. The distinction matters more than most patients realize, and section 2.4 returns to it. For now, understand that both are legitimate, both have limitations, and the choice affects how you should read the numbers.

2.2 Finding the Methane Line

Here is how to read your own result, step by step.

The following worked example uses a composite case.

Arden received a lactulose breath test result after months of constipation and afternoon bloating. The report had two curves plotted over time, one for hydrogen and one for methane, with the raw numbers listed in a table underneath. Arden had no idea which number mattered.

The first task is to locate the methane values across all the time points, not just one. The diagnostic rule for intestinal methanogen overgrowth is a methane level of ten parts per million or more at any point during the test (Rezaie et al., 2017; Pimentel et al., 2020). Read that carefully. It is not the peak, not the final value, not the average. It is any single reading that reaches ten. If Arden's methane touched twelve at the ninety minute mark and sat at six everywhere else, that single twelve is enough to meet the threshold. Methane behaves differently from hydrogen in this respect, and applying the hydrogen rules to the methane line is a common way to misread a report.

The second task is to check the baseline, the reading taken before Arden swallowed anything. With methane, a high baseline is itself meaningful. Because methanogens can colonize the whole intestinal tract and produce methane steadily rather than only in response to the test sugar, many methane dominant patients show elevated methane from the very first fasting measurement (Pimentel et al., 2020). Researchers have found that a single fasting methane measurement of ten or more correlates well with the fuller diagnosis, which is why some clinicians now pay close attention to that opening number (Takakura et al., 2022). Arden's baseline methane was eleven. It stayed elevated throughout. That flat, persistently high methane pattern is characteristic of overgrowth that has settled in for the long term.

The third task is to look at hydrogen in relation to methane. Arden's hydrogen was low across the board. This is not reassuring news that hides good methane news, it is part of the same story. Methanogens consume hydrogen to make methane, so a gut dominated by them often shows suppressed hydrogen and elevated methane at the same time (Villanueva-Millan et al., 2022). The low hydrogen is a fingerprint of the archaea at work, not evidence that little is wrong.

The complicating moment in Arden's case was the interpretation line printed at the bottom, which read hydrogen negative. Taken alone, that phrase might suggest a normal or near normal result, and a hurried reader could have stopped there and felt falsely reassured. Reading only the summary line, rather than the methane values across the full time course, would have missed the diagnosis entirely. The methane, elevated from baseline and never dropping below the threshold, was the finding that mattered.

2.3 What the Number Does and Does Not Tell You

Meeting the threshold tells you that methanogens are overgrown. It does not tell you how sick you will feel, and it does not by itself dictate your entire treatment. The relationship between the height of the methane number and the severity of symptoms is real but loose. Methane on breath testing is consistently associated with constipation across studies, and higher methane tends to track with slower transit and more constipation, but the correlation is not tight enough to read your suffering off the figure (Kunkel et al., 2011). Some people who scrape just over ten are debilitated. Others in the twenties are functioning.

This matters emotionally as much as clinically. Patients often fixate on the number, treating a twenty as catastrophic and a twelve as trivial, when in practice the number is a yes or no gate with a soft dial attached, not a precise measure of how bad things are. What the number gives you is entry into a specific diagnostic and treatment conversation, the one built around archaea and methane rather than around hydrogen. That conversation is the valuable thing, not the digit itself.

2.4 Glucose Versus Lactulose

The two sugars used in breath testing behave differently, and knowing which one you were given changes how you read the result.

Glucose is absorbed high in the small intestine, usually within the first stretch of it. Because it is taken up so quickly, a glucose test mainly interrogates the upper gut. Its strength is that a positive result is fairly specific, meaning a clear rise is unlikely to be a false alarm. Its weakness is that overgrowth lower down, further along the intestine, can be missed because the glucose has already been absorbed before it gets there (Saad & Chey, 2014).

Lactulose is not absorbed by humans at all. It travels the length of the small intestine and reaches the colon, which means it can detect overgrowth further down than glucose can. Its strength is broader reach. Its weakness is a higher rate of false positives and the complication that everyone's lactulose eventually reaches the colon, where colonic bacteria will ferment it and produce gas whether or not true overgrowth exists (Ghoshal, 2011; Saad & Chey, 2014).

For methane specifically, the choice is less fraught than for hydrogen, because a methane reading of ten or more at any point is the operative rule regardless of which sugar was used (Rezaie et al., 2017). Methanogens tend to produce methane fairly steadily rather than in a sharp substrate driven spike, so the persistent elevation that defines your subtype shows up on either test. Still, when you discuss your result with a clinician, knowing whether you had glucose or lactulose lets you weigh how much confidence to place in a borderline finding.

2.5 When the Test Misleads

No breath test is perfect, and methane results carry their own traps.

The first is preparation. In the day before a breath test you are usually asked to eat a restricted, low fermentation diet and then to fast overnight, and to avoid certain medications. Skipping the diet prep can inflate gas readings, because there is leftover fermentable food feeding the organisms. Certain medications, including motility drugs and recent antibiotics or laxatives, can distort the picture in either direction (Rezaie et al., 2017). If your preparation was imperfect, your result deserves to be read with more caution, and possibly repeated.

The second trap is treating a single test as the final word. Breath testing is a useful tool with genuine limitations, and clinicians who rely on it do so knowing it is an imperfect proxy for what is happening inside the gut (Ghoshal, 2011; Saad & Chey, 2014). A result that fits your symptom picture, constipation and bloating alongside elevated methane, is more trustworthy than a result that contradicts everything you are experiencing. When test and symptoms disagree sharply, the disagreement itself is information, and the answer is rarely to trust the paper over the person.

The following account is a composite, with details changed for anonymity.

Bellamy had put off testing for over a year, partly because of the cost and partly because she was afraid of what it would or would not show. When she finally did the test, she made two prep errors. She ate normally the day before because she had misread the instructions, and she took her usual fiber supplement that morning. Her methane came back at fourteen. Rather than accept the number at face value, her clinician noted the prep problems, acknowledged that the elevated fiber and food intake could have inflated the reading, and also noted that Bellamy's lifelong constipation and daily trapped bloating were exactly the clinical picture methane overgrowth produces. The decision was not to discard the result or to treat it as gospel, but to weigh it. The number was plausible because it agreed with everything Bellamy had lived with for years. A clean repeat test some weeks later, with proper preparation, came back at sixteen and settled the question. The lesson Bellamy took from it was that a breath test is evidence to be interpreted alongside her own experience, not a verdict handed down from a machine.

2.6 The Number Is a Starting Point

By now you can find the methane line on your own report, apply the ten parts per million any point rule correctly, read a low hydrogen result as part of the methane story rather than as reassurance, and judge how much weight your particular test deserves given how it was performed and whether it matches your symptoms. That is real fluency, and it puts you ahead of many patients who never get past the summary line.

Do this next. Take your own result, if you have one, and write down three things: the highest methane value and the time point it occurred, your fasting baseline methane, and whether your hydrogen was low, moderate, or high. Add one sentence on whether the result fits your lived symptoms or contradicts them. Those four pieces of information are what a good clinician will want, and having them ready turns your next appointment from a fishing expedition into a focused conversation. The number opened a door. The chapters ahead walk you through it, starting with the question of why methane, of all gases, is the one that stops your gut.

Chapter 3.0: Why Methane Slows Everything

Why are you constipated rather than loose? It is worth sitting with the strangeness of the question. Two people can have overgrowth in the same stretch of gut, driven by organisms fermenting the same food, and one ends up running to the bathroom while the other cannot go for days. The difference is not the amount of overgrowth or the severity of the dysbiosis. It is the gas. Hydrogen dominant overgrowth tends toward diarrhea. Methane dominant overgrowth tends toward constipation. And the reason is not a vague association or a statistical quirk. Methane does something physical and specific to the muscle of your intestine, and understanding that mechanism is what turns your constipation from an inexplicable curse into a solvable problem.

3.1 The Central Claim

The claim at the heart of this chapter is that methane is not a passive waste product drifting through your gut. It is biologically active, and its activity slows intestinal transit. This is not folklore. It was demonstrated directly in laboratory work showing that methane infused into intestinal tissue slowed the movement of contents through the bowel and changed the pattern of muscular contraction (Pimentel et al., 2006a). The finding reframed methane from a bystander gas into an active agent in the disease.

The consequence for you is that your constipation is, in a real sense, a symptom of methane exposure. The organisms in your gut are producing a gas that acts on your intestinal muscle in a way that makes the whole system move more slowly. This is why laxatives and fiber, which push against the symptom without touching the gas, so often disappoint. They are working downstream of the actual cause.

3.2 How the Slowing Happens

The mechanism operates at the level of the intestinal muscle and the nerves that coordinate it. Your gut moves its contents along through waves of coordinated contraction. Methane appears to interfere with the normal rhythm of these waves, dampening the forward propulsion that would ordinarily carry stool along and altering the local contractile activity of the small intestine (Pimentel et al., 2006a). The net effect is slower transit, both through the small bowel and through the colon.

This has been observed in patients, not just in the laboratory. Studies measuring how long it takes contents to travel through the gut have found that people with elevated methane show delayed transit through both the small intestine and the colon compared with those without it (Suri et al., 2018). The physiology demonstrated in tissue shows up as measurable slowness in real digestive tracts. And across the broader literature, the association between methane and constipation is one of the more consistent findings in this whole field, replicated across studies and summarized in systematic review (Kunkel et al., 2011).

There is a certain grim elegance to it. The archaea produce methane. The methane slows the gut. The slow gut is your constipation. Each link in that chain has been observed, and together they explain why your subtype produces the symptom it does.

3.3 The Self Reinforcing Loop

Here is where the story turns from unfortunate to genuinely stubborn. The slowing effect of methane does not just cause your constipation. It also helps sustain the overgrowth that produces the methane in the first place.

Your gut has a housekeeping function, a wave of muscular activity between meals that sweeps residual contents and microorganisms downstream and out. This sweeping wave, discussed in detail in Chapter 8, is one of the body's main defenses against overgrowth. When transit slows, that housekeeping falters. Organisms that would have been swept along instead linger, and organisms that linger have time to multiply. More methanogens mean more methane, and more methane means more slowing, which means still weaker housekeeping (Pimentel et al., 2020).

This is the loop, and it is the reason your condition resists simple solutions. Slow movement lets the organisms build. The organisms produce methane. The methane slows movement further. Round and round. It explains an experience that frustrates and confounds so many patients, the experience of killing the organisms with a course of treatment, feeling better briefly, and then relapsing within a few months. If the treatment addressed the organisms but left the slow motility untouched, the loop simply restarts. The gut is still sluggish, the housekeeping is still weak, and the overgrowth reestablishes itself in the hospitable conditions that never changed.

The following account is a composite, with details changed for anonymity.

Calloway had cleared his methane twice, once with antibiotics and once with a herbal protocol, and both times the constipation had returned within about four months. He had begun to think of himself as a hopeless case, someone whose gut simply regenerated the problem no matter what anyone did. What no one had explained to him was the loop. Both of his treatments had targeted the organisms and ignored the reason his gut had become hospitable to them, which was longstanding slow motility that predated the overgrowth. Each treatment knocked the methanogens back. Each time, his sluggish gut let them return. The turning point was not a stronger antimicrobial. It was the addition of a serious, sustained motility strategy alongside the treatment, so that after the organisms were reduced, the housekeeping wave was supported well enough to keep them from rebuilding. His improvement was not instant and it was not total, but for the first time the relapses stopped arriving on schedule.

Calloway's story illustrates the single most important practical implication of this chapter. Treating the overgrowth without treating the motility is treating half the loop. It can produce temporary relief, but temporary relief that reliably unravels is exactly what the loop predicts.

3.4 Correcting a Common Misreading

A misunderstanding worth heading off is the idea that if methane causes the constipation, then simply forcing the bowels to move, with strong enough laxatives, ought to solve everything. It does not, and the reason is instructive.

Laxatives act on the symptom. They can produce a bowel movement, sometimes several, but they do not reduce the methane, do not touch the archaea, and do not restore the housekeeping wave. You can force output while the underlying loop keeps turning, which is why so many methane patients describe being dependent on escalating doses that work less well over time. The laxative is bailing water out of a boat that is still taking it on. This does not mean laxatives have no place. Used thoughtfully and under guidance they can provide real relief while the actual causes are addressed. But relief is not repair, and mistaking one for the other keeps people cycling for years.

3.5 Two Paths From the Same Starting Point

The loop also explains why two patients who begin in similar places can diverge so sharply depending on whether the motility piece is addressed.

The following are composite cases.

Dune finished a course of combined treatment with her methane substantially reduced and her constipation eased for the first time in years. Understanding the loop, her clinician started her on a maintenance plan aimed squarely at motility, supporting the housekeeping wave between meals and spacing her eating to give the gut time to sweep. Her improvement was not perfect. She had setbacks, and one stretch of stress undid some of her progress. But the pattern of clockwork relapse every few months did not return, because the conditions that had allowed the overgrowth to rebuild had been changed.

Wren finished the same kind of treatment with the same initial result, methane down, constipation eased. But no one discussed motility with her, and she assumed the treatment had fixed the problem outright. She returned to her ordinary eating patterns and her ordinary grazing between meals, and her sluggish gut, never addressed, quietly went back to work. Within five months her methane and her symptoms had both returned. She concluded, understandably, that the treatment had failed. In truth the treatment had done its part. The loop had done the rest, in the space that the missing motility plan left open.

The two cases start identically and end differently, and the entire difference is whether the self reinforcing loop was interrupted or left intact. This is not a story about one patient being more diligent than the other. It is a story about whether the mechanism was understood and acted on.

3.6 A Loop You Can Interrupt

The methane in your gut is doing something concrete. It is slowing your intestinal muscle, delaying transit through both your small bowel and your colon, and in doing so it is weakening the very housekeeping function that would otherwise hold the overgrowth in check. That is why you are constipated rather than loose, and it is why treatment aimed only at the organisms tends to unravel.

The encouraging half of this picture is that a loop is precisely the kind of problem that offers more than one point of attack. You can reduce the organisms, which lowers methane production. You can support motility, which strengthens the housekeeping wave and closes the door that lets the overgrowth return. You can reduce the fermentable fuel that feeds the hydrogen the archaea depend on, which starves the cross feeding cycle upstream. Each of these is a lever, and the chapters ahead take them one at a time. Hold onto the shape of the loop as you read, because every treatment strategy in this book is, at bottom, an attempt to break it at one link or another. The first frustration to dismantle, the daily one, is the fiber and laxative advice that has failed you, and that is where the next chapter goes.

Chapter 4.0: The Fiber Paradox

Everyone knows that fiber helps constipation. It is the first advice a doctor gives, the first thing a search engine returns, the reflexive wisdom of every relative who has heard you complain. And for you, more fiber has quite possibly made things worse. Not neutral, not disappointing, actively worse. The bloating intensified, the fullness deepened, and the constipation you were trying to relieve did not budge. This is the fiber paradox, and living inside it, being told to do the one thing that reliably backfires, is one of the most disorienting experiences of methane dominant overgrowth. The contradiction is not in your head, and it is not a sign that your body is uniquely defective. It follows directly from the biology of the last two chapters.

4.1 The Problem Stated Plainly

The problem is this. Standard constipation advice assumes a gut that is short on bulk and moisture, where adding fermentable fiber gives the stool substance and draws in water, and things move. That advice is sound for ordinary constipation. It is close to counterproductive for methane dominant overgrowth, because your constipation is not primarily a bulk problem. It is a gas and motility problem.

When you add fermentable fiber to a gut colonized by overgrown organisms, you are feeding them. The bacteria ferment the fiber and release hydrogen. The methanogens consume that hydrogen and produce more methane (Villanueva-Millan et al., 2022). More methane means more of the transit slowing effect established in Chapter 3 (Pimentel et al., 2006a). So the fiber that was supposed to speed you up hands the archaea more raw material for the gas that slows you down. The bloating you feel after a high fiber meal is the fermentation happening in real time. This is the paradox in mechanical terms: in a methane dominant gut, some of the most recommended fibers are fuel for the problem.

4.2 Why the Usual Fixes Fall Short

The field's early answer to constipation, more fiber and more laxatives, falls short here for reasons that map onto the loop.

Fermentable fiber, as we have seen, can feed the overgrowth and increase gas. Bulk forming fiber supplements, the ones marketed hardest for constipation, are often the most fermentable and the most likely to worsen bloating in this population. Laxatives, meanwhile, act only on the symptom. They can produce a bowel movement without reducing methane, touching the archaea, or restoring the housekeeping wave, which means they provide output without repair (Pimentel et al., 2020). Patients frequently find themselves escalating laxative doses over time, chasing an effect that fades, because nothing about the underlying loop has changed.

None of this means fiber is your enemy or that you should strip it from your diet entirely. That overcorrection creates its own problems, which section 4.3 takes up. The point is narrower and more useful. The specific, high fermentation fibers that standard advice pushes hardest are frequently the wrong tool for a methane dominant gut, and reaching for more of them when they backfire is a predictable dead end.

4.3 The Pivot That Changes the Approach

What finally moves the needle is a reframe. Instead of asking how much fiber to add, you ask which fiber, in what amount, alongside what else. The goal shifts from bulking the stool to two things at once: reducing the fermentation that feeds methane, and supporting the motility that actually moves the gut.

This is a genuine tightrope, and it is worth naming honestly because the two aims pull against each other. You want to lower fermentable intake to reduce methane production. But you cannot strip fiber to zero, because some fiber and adequate fluid are part of what keeps stool moving at all, and a gut given nothing to work with becomes its own kind of constipated. The methane dominant patient has to reduce fermentation without starving the bowel, a balance that ordinary constipation advice never has to strike.

The practical shape of this balance is the subject of Chapter 9, which builds the eating approach in full. Here the point is conceptual. The pivot is away from the single dial of more fiber and toward a more careful adjustment: lowering the most fermentable fibers that spike gas, keeping or emphasizing gentler fibers and adequate fluid that support movement, and pairing all of it with the motility strategy that addresses the slowing directly. Fiber stops being a lever you crank up and becomes one input you tune among several.

The following account is a composite, with details changed for anonymity.

Ellis had done exactly what he was told. When his constipation worsened, he added a fiber supplement. When that did nothing, he doubled it. When the bloating became unbearable, he assumed he was not taking enough and pushed the dose higher still. By the time he sought help he was consuming a large daily quantity of a bulk forming fiber, more bloated than he had ever been, and no less constipated. The clinician who finally helped him did something that felt, to Ellis, completely backward. She had him reduce the fiber supplement rather than increase it, shifting toward smaller amounts of gentler, less fermentable fiber and adequate fluid, while addressing his methane and his motility directly. The bloating eased within a couple of weeks. His bowels, freed from the fermentation load that had been feeding the very gas slowing them, began to respond. Ellis described the experience as being told, for the first time, that the thing making him worse was the thing everyone had insisted would make him better.

4.4 Working It Through

To see how the reframe operates in practice, follow one worked example of the reasoning.

The following worked example uses a composite case.

Fallon presented with methane confirmed overgrowth, daily bloating that peaked in the evening, and constipation of several years' standing. She arrived convinced that her problem was insufficient fiber, because that was what she had always been told, and she wanted to know how much more to add.

Fallon's mental model was a bulk deficit, too little fiber, therefore add fiber. The clinician's first move was not to prescribe anything but to reframe the model. Fallon's constipation was downstream of methane and slow motility, not downstream of inadequate bulk. Adding fermentable fiber to that picture would feed the fermentation and raise the methane, which is the opposite of what she needed. This reframe had to come first, because every subsequent decision depended on it.

The obvious move, given that reframe, might seem to be cutting fiber drastically. The clinician did not do this. Stripping fiber and fluid too far would leave Fallon's already sluggish gut with nothing to move and could deepen the constipation from a different direction. The reasoning was to reduce the specific high fermentation fibers driving her evening bloating while preserving gentler fiber and ensuring adequate fluid. The aim was less fermentation, not less movement.

Fallon pushed back. She had read that a very low fermentation diet was the answer and wanted to eliminate as much fermentable food as possible, as fast as possible. The clinician declined to endorse an aggressive elimination, partly because such restriction is hard to sustain and partly because, in a constipated patient, cutting too much fermentable fiber at once can worsen the constipation before anything else has had time to work. Restriction was framed as a temporary tool with an endpoint, not a permanent way of eating, and it was paced rather than maximal.

The move that helped Fallon was not a bigger intervention in either direction, not more fiber and not brutal elimination. It was a tuned adjustment that respected both aims at once, lowering the fuel for methane while protecting the movement of the gut, and pairing the dietary change with treatment aimed at the organisms and the motility. The obvious approaches, add fiber or remove all fiber, were both rejected in favor of something more precise.

4.5 The Least Restriction That Works

A theme that will recur through the rest of this book, and one worth planting here, is that the goal is the least restriction that achieves the aim, not the most restriction you can tolerate. This matters practically and it matters psychologically.

Practically, over restriction backfires in a constipated gut, as Fallon's case showed. Cutting too much fermentable fiber can deepen constipation, and severe long term restriction risks poor nutrition and a diet so narrow it cannot be maintained. Psychologically, the endless shrinking of what feels safe to eat is its own harm, one that Chapter 12 addresses directly, because the anxiety that grows around food can outlast the gut symptoms that started it. A methane dominant patient who has been failed by fiber advice is understandably tempted to swing to the opposite extreme and eliminate everything, but maximal restriction is not the same as effective treatment, and it carries costs of its own.

4.6 Moving Is Not Fixing

The fiber paradox is not a mystery once you see the mechanism. In a methane dominant gut, the most recommended fibers feed the fermentation that produces the gas that slows your transit, which is why the standard advice can make you worse rather than better. And laxatives, however much relief they provide in the moment, produce movement without addressing methane, the archaea, or the housekeeping wave.

The reframe worth carrying out of this chapter is that in your condition, moving the bowels and fixing the problem are different things. A laxative moves. A more fermentable fiber may even move, at the cost of more gas. Neither fixes, because neither touches the loop. Fixing means reducing the organisms, supporting the motility, and tuning the diet to lower fermentation without starving the gut, all at once. That is more work than swallowing a fiber supplement, but it is work aimed at the actual causes rather than the surface. With the daily frustration of fiber and laxatives now accounted for, the book turns to the question that has probably haunted you longest: why the treatment that was supposed to fix all of this, the standard course everyone gets, did so little for you.

Chapter 5.0: Why Standard Treatment Underperforms

For most of the modern history of bacterial overgrowth, methane was an afterthought. Clinicians measured hydrogen, treated the overgrowth as a bacterial problem, and reached for the antibiotic that worked best against gut bacteria. Then a series of studies through the two thousands began to notice something inconvenient. The patients whose breath tests showed methane were not responding the way the hydrogen patients did. They stayed constipated. Their gas barely moved. The standard drug, effective and well tolerated for so many, was quietly failing a whole subgroup, and the field slowly worked out why. That story is worth understanding, because you are almost certainly a member of the subgroup, and the reason the standard treatment let you down is the same reason the field had to change its thinking.

5.1 The Era of One Drug for Everyone

The workhorse of bacterial overgrowth treatment is a nonabsorbable antibiotic that stays largely inside the gut, acting on the organisms there without being taken up into the rest of the body. Its record against ordinary, hydrogen dominant overgrowth is respectable, with eradication rates across studies that make it a sensible first choice for that population (Shah et al., 2013). For years it was prescribed more or less uniformly for anyone diagnosed with overgrowth, regardless of which gas their breath test showed. The label was overgrowth, the treatment was the standard antibiotic, and gas subtype was not part of the decision.

This worked acceptably for the hydrogen dominant majority and poorly for the methane dominant minority, but the failure was easy to miss at first. When a methane patient did not improve, the natural interpretation was that this particular patient was difficult, or noncompliant, or had some other problem layered on top. The idea that the drug itself was mismatched to the organism took time to surface, because it required first recognizing that the organism was not a bacterium at all.

5.2 The Observation That Forced a Change

The turning point came from studies that separated patients by the gas they produced and looked at how each group responded. When researchers examined methane positive patients specifically, the single standard antibiotic performed strikingly poorly. In the key study comparing treatments in methane positive patients, the standard nonabsorbable antibiotic alone eradicated methane in only about a quarter of subjects (Low et al., 2010). For a drug that performs respectably against hydrogen overgrowth, that is a dismal result, and it demanded an explanation.

A parallel line of work sharpened the picture. Researchers found that a different antibiotic, one with activity the standard drug lacked, improved constipation specifically in patients who had methane, and that the benefit depended on the presence of methane gas (Pimentel et al., 2006b). In other words, the drug helped precisely the methane patients and did so in a way tied to the methane itself. The gas was not incidental to treatment response. It was central to it.

Put together, these findings said something the old one drug approach could not accommodate. Methane patients were a distinct group. They responded differently to different drugs. And the standard antibiotic, prescribed reflexively for everyone, was close to the wrong tool for them.

5.3 The Biological Reason

The explanation, once the field arrived at it, connects directly to Chapter 1. The organisms producing methane are archaea, not bacteria, and archaea differ from bacteria in the very structures that antibiotics target. Many antibacterial drugs work by attacking features specific to bacterial cells. Archaea, belonging to a separate domain of life, do not have those features in the same form, which makes them intrinsically less susceptible to drugs designed for bacteria (Pimentel et al., 2020).

This is why the standard single antibiotic disappoints against methane. It is not that your case is unusually stubborn or that the drug is weak. It is that the drug was engineered for a target you are not primarily carrying. Asking it to clear an archaeal overgrowth is a little like using a key cut for one lock on a different lock entirely. It may rattle something, but it will not turn.

There is a further layer, the cross feeding relationship from Chapter 1. Because methanogens depend on hydrogen produced by bacteria, an effective strategy has to address both partners, cutting the hydrogen supply and targeting the archaea themselves. A single drug aimed at one part of that relationship leaves the other intact, which is part of why combination approaches, developed next in Chapter 6, outperform any single agent (Low et al., 2010). The old approach failed not only because it targeted the wrong organism but because it targeted only one side of a two sided problem.

The following account is a composite, with details changed for anonymity.

Briar had been treated for overgrowth four separate times over two years, each time with the same standard antibiotic, each time by a clinician acting on the diagnosis in her notes rather than the gas on her breath test. Her methane was substantial and had never been the focus of a single treatment decision. She had come to believe that her body simply defeated antibiotics, a belief that had hardened into a quiet hopelessness. When a gastroenterologist finally looked at the actual breath test rather than the diagnosis code, the picture reorganized in an afternoon. Briar had never received a treatment aimed at archaea. She had received, four times, a treatment aimed at bacteria, in a gut whose problem was not primarily bacterial. Her lack of response had never been resistance. It had been a mismatch, repeated. The relief of that reframe, she said afterward, was almost as large as the eventual physical improvement, because for two years she had been carrying the wrong story about her own body.

5.4 What the History Reveals

The arc from one drug for everyone to gas specific treatment is more than a historical curiosity. It reveals something about how you should understand your own treatment failures.

If the standard antibiotic did little for you, the most likely explanation is not that you are among the unfortunate few for whom nothing works. It is that you received a treatment developed and validated primarily for a different gas and a different organism. The history of this field is, in part, the history of clinicians realizing that a single label was hiding two different diseases, and that treating them the same way guaranteed that one of the two groups would keep failing. You are, in all probability, a member of the group the old approach was never built to help.

This reframe has a practical edge. When you sit with a clinician, the fact that a single standard antibiotic underperformed is not evidence that you are treatment resistant. It is evidence, entirely consistent with the literature, that your overgrowth is archaeal and needs an approach designed for archaea. That distinction changes what should happen next, and it is worth stating clearly rather than letting a string of past failures be misread as a property of your body.

5.5 Same Diagnosis, Different Paths

The way a single label can send two patients down different roads is worth making concrete.

The following are composite cases.

Cypress had a hydrogen dominant breath test, brisk early rise, negligible methane, and loose stools. Treated with the standard nonabsorbable antibiotic, he improved. The drug matched his organism, a bacterium, and his gas, hydrogen. His course did roughly what the literature predicts for that population (Shah et al., 2013). His overgrowth still had underlying causes that needed attention, but the initial treatment was appropriate and effective.

Garnet carried the same diagnosis on paper, overgrowth, but her breath test showed low hydrogen and high methane, and her dominant symptom was constipation. Given the identical drug Cypress received, because the notes said the same word, she barely responded. Her methane was archaeal, and the drug was built for bacteria. Only when her treatment was redesigned around the combined approach for methane, described in the next chapter, did she begin to change (Low et al., 2010; Pimentel et al., 2006b).

Cypress and Garnet were filed under one label and needed two treatments. The label predicted their prescription, and the prescription predicted that one of them would fail. Nothing about Garnet was harder to treat in principle. She simply needed a treatment aimed at her actual organism, and the shared label had obscured that need.

5.6 Built for the Wrong Target

The standard treatment underperformed for you because it was built for the wrong target. Developed and validated primarily against hydrogen dominant, bacterial overgrowth, it does respectable work in that population and close to the wrong work in yours, because your overgrowth is archaeal, your organisms belong to a separate domain of life, and the drug's mechanism aims at bacterial structures your methanogens do not share in the same way. The field learned this the hard way, by noticing that methane patients kept failing a treatment that should have worked, and by tracing that failure to the biology underneath the shared label.

The synthesis to carry forward is that treatment failure with a single standard antibiotic is not a statement about your resilience. It is a statement about matching. The right question is not why nothing works for you, because that framing is almost certainly false. The right question is what a treatment designed for archaea and their hydrogen supplying partners looks like. The field has an answer, developed over the same years it spent recognizing the problem, and that answer is where the next chapter goes.

Chapter 6.0: The Combined Approach Explained

A patient sits across from a gastroenterologist, breath test in hand, methane clearly above threshold, and asks the obvious question. If one antibiotic did not work, what will? The clinician explains that for methane, the evidence points not to a stronger single drug but to two drugs used together, each doing a different job, and that this combination outperforms either one alone. The patient nods, then hesitates, then asks the question that this entire chapter exists to answer. Why two? What is the second one actually for? This chapter walks through the logic of the combined antimicrobial approach in enough detail that you can hold exactly that conversation, understanding not just that two drugs are used but why the pairing works.

Before going further, one boundary must be absolutely clear. Everything in this chapter is explanation, not instruction. The medications discussed are prescription drugs with real risks, and the combined regimens are decisions for a prescriber who has examined you and knows your history. Nothing here is a protocol to attempt on your own, and antibiotics obtained or dosed without medical supervision can cause serious harm. Read this chapter to understand the reasoning, so that you can participate in the decision, never to bypass the person qualified to make it.

6.1 What the Combined Approach Involves

The combined antimicrobial approach for methane overgrowth pairs two antibiotics that do different things. The first is the nonabsorbable antibiotic familiar from ordinary overgrowth treatment, the one that acts broadly on gut bacteria. The second is a different antibiotic with activity the first one lacks, added specifically because it improves outcomes in methane positive patients (Low et al., 2010; Pimentel et al., 2006b).

The reasoning behind the pairing returns to the cross feeding relationship. Methanogens are archaea that depend on hydrogen produced by ordinary bacteria. If you target only the archaea, you leave their hydrogen supply intact. If you target only the bacteria, you cut the hydrogen supply but leave the archaea themselves in place. The logic of the combination is to do both at once, reducing the bacterial hydrogen production that feeds the methanogens while also directly targeting the methane producing organisms (Low et al., 2010). One drug addresses the supply, the other addresses the consumers, and together they attack both sides of the relationship a single drug can only half address.

This is why, for methane, combination therapy is the approach the evidence supports, while for hydrogen dominant overgrowth a single drug is often sufficient. The two conditions call for different strategies because they involve different organisms in different relationships.

6.2 What the Evidence Shows

The strongest single piece of evidence for the combined approach comes from a study that compared three treatments in methane positive patients: the standard nonabsorbable antibiotic alone, the second antibiotic alone, and the two combined (Low et al., 2010). The results were clear in a way that reshaped practice. Each drug alone eradicated methane in only a minority of patients, roughly a quarter to a third. The combination did substantially better. Among patients who had failed to clear their methane on the standard antibiotic alone, a majority went on to normalize their breath test when the second drug was added (Low et al., 2010).

Those figures deserve to be stated carefully, because inflated versions circulate widely. What the study supports is that combination therapy clearly outperformed either single agent, and that most prior non responders improved when the second drug was added. You will encounter higher, rounder numbers quoted confidently on websites and in marketing, and some of those trace to different or secondary datasets rather than to this study. The honest summary is that the combination works meaningfully better than one drug, that this is well established for methane, and that the precise eradication percentage varies by source and should not be oversold.

It is also worth being honest about the quality of the evidence base as a whole. The professional guidelines that recommend treating methane overgrowth rate much of the underlying evidence as low or very low quality, reflecting the reliance on smaller studies, retrospective reviews, and heterogeneous methods (Pimentel et al., 2020). This does not mean the combined approach is unfounded. It means the confidence behind it is moderate rather than absolute, and a good clinician will hold it that way, as a well supported strategy rather than a guarantee.

6.3 Where It Breaks Down

Combination therapy is more effective than single drug treatment for methane, but more effective is not the same as reliably curative, and the approach has real limits worth understanding.

The first limit is relapse. Even when the combination successfully clears methane, the overgrowth can return, sometimes within months, because clearing the organisms does not by itself repair the slow motility that let them accumulate in the first place (Pimentel et al., 2020). This is the loop from Chapter 3 reasserting itself. Treatment that reduces the organisms without addressing the motility is treating half the problem, which is why Chapter 8 argues that motility support is not optional maintenance but part of the core strategy.

The second limit is the second drug itself. The additional antibiotic added for methane is a broad acting agent, and broad acting antibiotics carry more collateral effect on the wider gut community than the narrowly focused nonabsorbable drug does. This is one of the trade offs a prescriber weighs, and it is a legitimate reason the decision belongs to a clinician rather than to a website. There are alternative second agents and alternative regimens, and which one fits depends on your history, your other conditions, and your prescriber's judgment. The existence of these trade offs is precisely why this chapter refuses to hand you a regimen.

The third limit is that antibiotics do nothing about the reasons your gut became hospitable to overgrowth. If an underlying driver, a motility disorder, a structural issue, a consequence of another condition, remains unaddressed, treatment will keep having to be repeated. Chapter 10 takes up the search for those drivers directly.

6.4 Diagnosing the Disappointments

When combination therapy underperforms, the reasons usually fall into recognizable patterns, and understanding them helps you and your clinician respond rather than simply conclude that nothing works.

The following is a composite case; identifying details have been changed.

Indigo, in her late thirties, had confirmed methane overgrowth with a breath test methane of nineteen and years of constipation and evening bloating. She had responded partially to a single antibiotic in the past, with brief relief followed by return of symptoms. She presented after a course of combination therapy that had helped less than she hoped. Her constipation had eased for perhaps six weeks and then crept back, though not quite to its former severity. She was discouraged and half convinced she was untreatable.

Two things stood out on analysis. First, the combination had in fact worked, in the sense that her symptoms had genuinely improved before returning, which suggested the organisms had been reduced. Second, nothing in her treatment had addressed her motility, and her history, including a long standing tendency to slow transit that predated the overgrowth, pointed to exactly the kind of sluggish housekeeping that lets methane rebuild. The relapse was not evidence of treatment failure. It was evidence of the loop closing again in the absence of a motility plan.

Rather than reaching immediately for another, stronger course of antibiotics, the clinician added a sustained motility strategy after the antimicrobial treatment, aimed at supporting the between meal housekeeping wave, along with attention to the dietary fermentation load. The antimicrobial work was treated as one phase, not the whole treatment. At follow up several months later, Indigo's improvement had held better than after any previous treatment, though it was not complete and required ongoing attention. She still had difficult stretches. What had changed was the pattern of reliable relapse, which had not returned on its old schedule.

> **Teaching Point:** *Partial relapse after effective combination therapy usually points to unaddressed motility, not to a failed drug. The antimicrobial phase reduces the organisms. The maintenance phase keeps them from rebuilding. Treating the first as the entire treatment predicts exactly the relapse Indigo experienced.*

6.5 A Harder Application

Not every case resolves as tidily as adding a motility plan, and it helps to see a more complicated one.

The following account is a composite, with details changed for anonymity.

Kestrel had methane overgrowth alongside another significant medical condition that affected his gut, which complicated every treatment decision. The combined antibiotic approach that might have been straightforward in a simpler patient carried more risk for him, because one of the drugs interacted with his broader situation and because his underlying condition kept regenerating the conditions for overgrowth. His clinician could not simply run the standard combination and add motility support. The decision required weighing the benefit of clearing his methane against the risks the combination posed given everything else, considering alternative agents, and accepting that treatment would likely need to be an ongoing management effort rather than a one time fix.

Kestrel's outcome was genuinely mixed. He improved, but incompletely, and he needed periodic re treatment as his underlying condition dictated. His case illustrates something the neat studies can obscure, that real patients arrive with histories and comorbidities that turn a clean protocol into a series of judgment calls. It also illustrates, again, why this chapter will not hand anyone a regimen. The reasoning is teachable. The specific decision is not, because it depends on details only a clinician examining you can see.

6.6 A Conversation Not a Prescription

The combined antimicrobial approach for methane rests on a coherent logic. Methanogens are archaea that live on hydrogen supplied by bacteria, so an effective attack targets both, cutting the supply with one drug and hitting the archaea with another, which is why two drugs used together outperform either alone in methane positive patients (Low et al., 2010; Pimentel et al., 2006b). The evidence supports the combination clearly, even as the professional guidelines rate the overall evidence base as low quality and honest sources decline to oversell the exact numbers (Pimentel et al., 2020).

Take this into your next appointment as questions, not as a plan. Ask whether your methane result supports a combined approach rather than a single drug. Ask what second agent your clinician would consider and why. Ask how the plan addresses relapse and motility, not just the immediate overgrowth. Ask what the trade offs of the second antibiotic are for you specifically. Those questions mark you as an informed patient collaborating in a decision, which is exactly the position this chapter is meant to put you in. The prescription is the clinician's to write. The understanding is yours to bring, and it changes the quality of the decision that gets made. With the pharmaceutical approach mapped, the next chapter turns to the question so many patients ask next, whether herbal antimicrobials are a real alternative or a distraction.

Chapter 7.0: The Herbal Question

I will admit something that a lot of writers in this space will not. The evidence on herbal antimicrobials for methane overgrowth is thinner and messier than either their fiercest advocates or their loudest skeptics let on, and anyone who tells you the question is settled, in either direction, is selling you a position rather than the truth. The honest picture is more interesting than the tribal one. There is a real study worth knowing about, real limitations worth naming, and a genuine disagreement among serious people about where herbal options belong. This chapter presents that disagreement fairly, because you deserve to make your own decision from the actual state of the evidence rather than from marketing on one side or reflexive dismissal on the other.

7.1 The Disagreement Stated Fairly

The disagreement is not really about whether herbal antimicrobials do anything. It is about how much weight the evidence can bear and where these agents sit relative to prescription treatment.

On one side are clinicians and patients who see herbal antimicrobials as a legitimate, evidence supported option, sometimes preferable to antibiotics for their gentler profile, and point to a study suggesting comparable effectiveness. On the other side are clinicians who regard the evidence as too thin and too poorly controlled to justify placing herbals alongside pharmaceutical treatment, and who worry that the natural framing lends these products an undeserved air of safety. Both positions are held by serious people, and both have something real underneath them. The task is not to declare a winner but to give each side its strongest case and then show you where the evidence actually runs out.

7.2 The Strongest Case for Herbals

The single most cited piece of evidence for herbal antimicrobials in overgrowth is a study that compared a herbal antimicrobial protocol against the standard prescription antibiotic and found the herbal approach to be at least as effective for clearing overgrowth on breath testing (Chedid et al., 2014). This is a real, published finding, and it is the backbone of the case for herbals. Advocates point out, reasonably, that if a herbal protocol performs comparably to the prescription standard, it deserves a place at the table, particularly for patients who cannot tolerate or prefer to avoid antibiotics.

There is also a plausible biological rationale for at least some herbal agents against methanogens specifically. Certain plant derived compounds, including one derived from garlic, have been proposed to act against the archaea that produce methane, though the evidence for this is preliminary and drawn largely from laboratory and animal work rather than from studies in people. This matters because, as Chapter 1 established, methanogens are archaea and resist many standard antibiotics. An agent with genuine anti archaeal activity is at least aimed at the right kind of organism.

The advocates' strongest overall point is a practical one. For a patient who has failed or cannot take the prescription route, a herbal protocol with a supporting study and a plausible mechanism is not nothing. It is a reasonable option to discuss, not a fringe indulgence.

7.3 The Strongest Case for Caution

The case against leaning on herbals is equally worth stating on its own terms, because it is not mere prejudice against anything natural.

The evidence base is genuinely thin. The comparison study, while real and worth citing, is a single study of modest size, and it did not separate patients cleanly by gas subtype in the way a methane specific reader would want (Chedid et al., 2014). Building a treatment philosophy on one modest study is exactly the kind of overreach that the low quality evidence problem, flagged throughout this book, warns against. The broader herbal literature for overgrowth is small, variable in quality, and short on the kind of rigorous, replicated trials that would let anyone speak with confidence.

There is also the safety framing problem. The word natural does a great deal of quiet persuasive work, implying gentleness and safety that the actual products may not warrant. Herbal antimicrobials are biologically active compounds. They can have side effects, interact with medications, and vary enormously in formulation and dose between products, with little of the standardization that governs prescription drugs. A patient who assumes a herbal protocol is inherently safe because it is not a drug is making an assumption the evidence does not support.

Finally, there is the commercial context. Herbal protocols are frequently sold as part of paid programs and supplement packages, and the financial incentive to promote them is substantial. This does not make them ineffective, but it does mean the enthusiasm you encounter online is not disinterested, and some patients have been both physically harmed and financially exploited by unregulated practitioners promoting aggressive supplement regimens. Skepticism in this context is not closed mindedness. It is appropriate caution about a lightly regulated market.

7.4 What the Evidence Actually Shows

Strip away both the marketing and the dismissal, and here is what can honestly be said.

There is one reasonable quality study suggesting a herbal antimicrobial protocol can perform comparably to the standard prescription antibiotic for clearing overgrowth (Chedid et al., 2014). There is a plausible biological rationale for targeting methanogens specifically, though direct evidence that particular agents clear them in people remains preliminary. And there is a great deal that is not known, including how herbal protocols perform specifically in methane dominant patients, how they compare to the combination approach that is the real standard for methane rather than to a single antibiotic, how different formulations and doses compare, and what their long term safety profile is.

The evidence supports treating herbal antimicrobials as a plausible option worth discussing with a knowledgeable clinician, especially for patients who cannot use antibiotics. It does not support treating them as an established equal to pharmaceutical treatment for methane, and it certainly does not support the confident, curative claims that surround them commercially. That is an unsatisfying answer if you wanted a verdict, but it is the honest one, and an honest uncertain answer serves you better than a confident wrong one.

7.5 Two Reasonable Choices

Because the evidence genuinely permits more than one reasonable choice, it helps to see two patients making different decisions, both defensibly.

The following are composite cases.

Joss had a serious adverse reaction to an antibiotic years earlier and was deeply reluctant to take another. Working with a clinician who knew the evidence, she chose a supervised herbal antimicrobial protocol for her methane overgrowth, understanding that the evidence was limited but reasoning that, given her history, a plausible option with a supporting study was preferable to a drug she feared. Her result was partial. Her methane came down and her symptoms improved, though not completely, and she needed to pair the approach with motility support to hold the gains. Her choice was reasonable given her circumstances, and it was made with open eyes about the uncertainty.

Nyx, facing the same diagnosis without any history of drug intolerance, chose the combination antibiotic approach because he wanted the treatment with the strongest evidence for methane specifically, and the herbal evidence, as his clinician explained, did not yet match it for his subtype. His result was also partial, good initial response, some relapse, improvement with added motility work. His choice was also reasonable, made for different but equally valid reasons.

The contrast is the point. Joss and Nyx reached opposite decisions from the same evidence, and neither was wrong, because the evidence permits both when weighed against individual circumstances. What would have been wrong is either patient being told there was only one legitimate answer, or being sold a herbal protocol as a guaranteed cure, or being dismissed for considering one at all.

7.6 Options Without Tribes

The herbal question does not resolve cleanly, and pretending otherwise would betray the honesty this book is trying to keep. What can be said is bounded and fair. There is a real study supporting comparable effectiveness for a herbal protocol against the standard antibiotic, a plausible rationale for some agents against methanogens, and a substantial amount that remains unknown, particularly for the methane subtype specifically (Chedid et al., 2014). Herbal antimicrobials are a plausible option to discuss, not an established equal to pharmaceutical treatment, and the natural label should never be mistaken for a safety guarantee.

Where this leaves you is with a decision to make rather than a rule to follow, and that is appropriate given the state of the evidence.

The useful stance is options without tribes. Neither the camp that treats herbals as obviously superior nor the camp that dismisses them entirely is reasoning from the actual evidence, which is more modest and more uncertain than either admits. Bring the question to a clinician who knows the literature, weigh it against your own history and tolerances, and be as skeptical of confident herbal cure claims as you are of any other oversold promise. One thing both the pharmaceutical and herbal paths share, whichever you choose, is that neither works durably without the piece the next chapter argues is the true center of the whole effort, the restoration of your gut's own movement.

Chapter 8.0: Motility Is the Whole Game

Here is a figure that should stop you. Even after a course of treatment successfully clears the overgrowth, a large share of patients relapse, sometimes within a few months, and the recurrence has been observed to climb over the year that follows (Pimentel et al., 2020). That number does not fit the story most people are told about overgrowth, which is that you take the treatment, you clear the organisms, and you are better. If clearing the organisms were the whole answer, the relapse rate would be low. It is not low, and the reason it is not low is the single most important practical fact in this book. The organisms are not the root problem. The gut that let them accumulate is. Until that gut is addressed, treatment keeps working temporarily and failing predictably.

8.1 The Problem of Reliable Relapse

The problem is stark once you name it plainly. Patients complete effective treatment, feel real relief, and then watch their symptoms return on a schedule, three months, four months, six months, again and again. Each relapse feels like a personal failure or a sign of an especially stubborn case, when in fact it is the expected result of treating only half the condition.

The half that gets treated is the overgrowth itself, the organisms and the methane they produce. The half that gets ignored is the reason the overgrowth was able to establish in the first place, which for most methane patients is slow motility, a gut that does not move its contents along briskly enough to keep organisms from accumulating. When treatment reduces the organisms but leaves the sluggish gut unchanged, the sluggish gut simply repopulates. The relapse is not bad luck. It is the loop from Chapter 3 completing another circuit in the space that the missing motility work left open.

8.2 The Housekeeping Wave

To understand why motility is the whole game, you need to understand a specific feature of how your gut works between meals, a feature that is central to preventing overgrowth and that goes wrong in most methane patients.

When you are not eating, your small intestine performs a periodic sweeping action, a wave of muscular contraction that travels down its length and pushes residual food particles and microorganisms ahead of it, clearing the small bowel and moving its contents onward. This wave, called the migrating motor complex, functions like a housekeeping cycle, running during the gaps between meals when the gut is empty (Ghoshal, 2011). It is one of the body's primary defenses against overgrowth, because it prevents organisms from settling and multiplying in the small intestine by regularly sweeping them out.

The finding that ties this directly to your condition is that patients with overgrowth have been shown to have a reduced frequency of this housekeeping wave (Pimentel et al., 2002). Their sweeping cycle runs less often, which means their small intestine is cleared less effectively, which means organisms have more opportunity to accumulate. This is not a minor detail. It is arguably the central mechanical failure behind overgrowth in general, and it is worsened, in your case, by the methane that slows the gut further, deepening the very deficit that let the methanogens flourish. A weak housekeeping wave allows overgrowth. Overgrowth produces methane. Methane weakens the housekeeping wave. The loop again.

8.3 The Pivot Toward Prevention

What changed the approach to relapse was the recognition that if a weak housekeeping wave allows overgrowth, then strengthening or supporting that wave should help prevent it from returning. This shifted the goal of treatment from a single act of clearance to an ongoing effort at maintenance, with motility support at its center.

The evidence for this pivot is meaningful. In a study of relapse prevention, low doses of agents that stimulate the housekeeping wave, taken at night, delayed the return of symptoms after treatment compared with what happened without them (Pimentel et al., 2009). The logic is exactly what the housekeeping wave account predicts. Support the sweeping cycle, and the small intestine is cleared more effectively between meals, and the overgrowth takes longer to reestablish. Agents used this way are called prokinetics, meaning they promote gut movement, and they act not by killing organisms but by supporting the motility that keeps organisms from accumulating (Pimentel et al., 2009).

This reframes the entire treatment sequence. The antimicrobial phase, whether pharmaceutical or herbal, reduces the existing overgrowth. The motility phase that follows aims to keep it from coming back. Treating the first phase as the whole treatment is the mistake that produces the relapse figure this chapter opened with. The prevention phase is not an optional extra for the especially cautious. It is the part of the strategy that addresses the actual root of the problem.

8.4 Supporting Motility in Practice

There is more than one way to support the housekeeping wave, and the details belong to a clinician, but the categories are worth understanding.

Prescription prokinetics are medications that stimulate gut motility, used at low doses, often at night, to support the between meal sweeping cycle after treatment (Pimentel et al., 2009). Which agent suits a given patient depends on their history and other conditions, and these are prescription decisions. There are also gentler, non prescription approaches sometimes used to support motility, and lifestyle measures that matter regardless of medication.

Among the lifestyle measures, meal spacing is one of the most important and least appreciated. The housekeeping wave runs during the gaps between meals, when the gut is empty. Every time you eat, you interrupt it, because the gut switches from housekeeping mode to digestion mode. A person who grazes continuously, snacking every hour or two through the day, gives the housekeeping wave almost no chance to run. Leaving meaningful gaps between meals, and a longer overnight fast, creates the empty stretches during which the sweeping cycle can do its work. This is not a dramatic intervention, but it is a real one, and it costs nothing.

The following account is a composite, with details changed for anonymity.

Linden had cleared her methane and, understanding at last that motility was the point, took the maintenance phase seriously. She worked with her clinician on a prokinetic approach and, on her own, restructured her eating. She had been a lifelong grazer, someone who ate small amounts more or less constantly, and she had never connected that habit to her gut. She began leaving real gaps between meals, three or four hours, and lengthening her overnight fast. The change was not comfortable at first, and it did not produce overnight transformation. But over months her pattern of relapse, which had been almost seasonal in its regularity, loosened its grip. She still had difficult periods, particularly under stress, but the reliable return of her symptoms every few months did not recur. What had changed, she realized, was that for the first time her gut was being given the empty time it needed to clean itself.

8.5 Two Endings to the Same Treatment

The difference the maintenance phase makes is best seen in two patients whose antimicrobial treatment went equally well.

The following are composite cases.

Oakley finished combination treatment with his methane cleared and his constipation eased. His clinician framed the maintenance phase as central, not optional, and started him on a motility supporting plan with attention to meal spacing. His path was not smooth. He had a relapse after a stressful stretch and needed his plan adjusted. But across the following year his condition was manageable in a way it had never been, because the underlying motility deficit was being addressed continuously rather than ignored.

Rumi finished the same treatment with the same good initial result. But her maintenance was an afterthought, mentioned briefly and never built into a real plan, and she understood the cleared methane as the end of her treatment. She resumed her ordinary continuous grazing and took nothing to support her motility. Her sluggish gut, entirely unaddressed, went quietly back to accumulating organisms. Within about five months her methane and her constipation had both returned, and she entered the cycle of re treatment that so many patients know, clearing and relapsing and clearing again.

The treatments were identical and the endings diverged, and the whole of the difference was whether the motility deficit that underlies the condition was treated as the center of the effort or as a footnote to it. Rumi was not less diligent than Oakley about the part she was told mattered. She was simply never told that the part that actually mattered was the part that came after the antibiotics.

8.6 Where Durable Change Lives

The relapse figure that opened this chapter is not a mystery and not a verdict on your resilience. It is the predictable consequence of treating overgrowth as though clearing the organisms were the whole job. The organisms accumulate because the gut's housekeeping wave, its between meal sweeping cycle, runs too weakly to keep them out, and that weak wave is deepened by the very methane the overgrowth produces. Clear the organisms and leave the wave weak, and the organisms return. This is why a majority of patients can relapse after successful treatment, and why the number should reframe how you think about the entire effort (Pimentel et al., 2020; Pimentel et al., 2009).

The synthesis to carry forward is that durable change does not live in the antimicrobial phase, however important that phase is. It lives in the maintenance that follows, in supporting the motility that keeps the overgrowth from rebuilding. The antibiotics or herbs buy you a cleared gut. The motility work is what lets you keep it. Any treatment plan that ends when the antimicrobials end is a plan built to relapse, and recognizing that is the difference between cycling for years and actually moving forward. The next chapter takes up the daily companion to motility work, the eating approach that lowers the fermentation feeding your methane without starving the gut you are trying to keep moving.

Chapter 9.0: Eating Without Endless Restriction

There is a note taped inside a kitchen cabinet in more homes than you would guess, a handwritten list of forbidden foods that has grown longer over the months until it covers most of what a person used to eat. Each item was added after a bad day, a swollen afternoon, a night of discomfort traced back to something eaten. The list represents an entirely understandable response to a gut that has become unpredictable, and it is also, quite often, making things worse. This chapter is about replacing that ever growing list of forbidden foods with something more precise and more sustainable, an eating approach that lowers the fermentation feeding your methane without shrinking your diet to a punishing handful of safe items.

9.1 What This Approach Involves

The eating approach for methane overgrowth has two aims that must be held together, and it is defined as much by what it refuses to do as by what it does.

The first aim is to reduce fermentation. The methanogens producing your methane depend on hydrogen, and that hydrogen comes largely from bacteria fermenting certain carbohydrates in your food. Reduce the most fermentable of those carbohydrates, and you reduce the hydrogen supply, which starves the cross feeding cycle that produces methane (Villanueva-Millan et al., 2022). This is the rationale behind the low fermentation eating patterns commonly used for overgrowth.

The second aim, easy to forget and vital for you specifically, is to keep the gut moving. You are constipated. Strip fermentable fiber and fluid too aggressively, and you can deepen the constipation, because a gut given too little to work with slows further. The methane patient cannot simply minimize everything fermentable the way a diarrhea dominant patient might, because the constipation sets a floor below which restriction becomes counterproductive.

The whole approach lives in the tension between these two aims. Lower fermentation enough to reduce methane, but not so much that you worsen the constipation or make the diet impossible to sustain. This is why the governing principle of this chapter is the least restriction that works, not the most restriction you can bear.

9.2 Working Through the Reasoning

To see how this balance is struck, follow the reasoning in a single worked example.

The following worked example uses a composite case.

Solstice arrived with confirmed methane overgrowth, evening bloating, and constipation, and with a food list so long she was eating perhaps a dozen items on rotation. She wanted to know what else to cut, because cutting was the only tool she had.

The clinician's first move was to reverse Solstice's question. She was asking what more to eliminate. The better question was what could be added back safely, because her extreme restriction was itself part of the problem, worsening her constipation by depriving her gut of fiber and variety, and feeding a growing anxiety around food. The reframe mattered because every subsequent step depended on abandoning the more is better model of restriction.

Rather than treating all her forbidden foods as equally guilty, the clinician worked to identify which foods actually drove Solstice's symptoms. Much of her list had been assembled from single bad days and coincidence, not from any consistent pattern. The high fermentation foods most likely to be feeding her methane were a smaller set than her list implied. Targeting that smaller set, rather than the sprawling list, was the aim. The plan reduced the specific high fermentation foods most associated with her bloating while deliberately preserving gentler fiber and adequate fluid to protect her already sluggish transit. This is the balance in action, lowering the fuel for methane while keeping the gut supplied enough to move.

Solstice wanted to do a maximal elimination immediately, convinced that faster and stricter was better. The clinician declined. Aggressive elimination is hard to sustain, risks worsening constipation by cutting too much fiber at once, and tends to intensify food anxiety rather than relieve it. Restriction was framed as a temporary, targeted tool with a planned endpoint and a reintroduction phase, not as a permanent contraction of her diet. The obvious move, cut more and faster, was rejected in favor of a paced, bounded reduction.

What helped Solstice was not another item on the forbidden list. It was a smaller, smarter reduction paired with the beginning of expansion, restriction treated as a phase rather than a way of life. The reasoning refused both extremes, the sprawling avoidance she arrived with and the maximal elimination she requested, in favor of a targeted middle that respected both her methane and her constipation.

9.3 Where It Breaks Down

The eating approach fails in recognizable ways, and knowing them helps you avoid them.

It breaks down when restriction has no endpoint. A low fermentation diet is a tool for a phase of treatment, meant to reduce methane while other work proceeds, not a permanent way of eating. Left open ended, it narrows the diet indefinitely, risks nutritional inadequacy, and becomes progressively harder to sustain. The absence of a planned reintroduction is one of the most common ways this approach goes wrong.

It breaks down when restriction is too aggressive for a constipated gut. Cutting fermentable fiber too far can worsen the very constipation you are trying to relieve, which is a trap specific to the methane patient and one that a diarrhea oriented overgrowth diet will not warn you about.

And it breaks down when it is done in isolation. Diet reduces the fermentation feeding methane, but it does not clear an established overgrowth on its own and does not repair motility. Patients who pin all their hope on diet, expecting food changes alone to resolve the condition, are usually disappointed, because diet is one lever among the several this book has laid out, not the whole machine.

9.4 Reintroduction and the Endpoint

Because the diet is a tool with an end, the reintroduction phase is not an afterthought but a planned part of the approach.

Once the overgrowth has been treated and methane reduced, foods that were restricted are reintroduced gradually, both to widen the diet back toward normal and to learn which foods a person actually tolerates now versus which were only problems while the overgrowth was active. Many foods that caused trouble during active overgrowth are tolerated fine once the methane is down and the motility supported, which means permanent avoidance of them was never necessary. Reintroduction is how you find that out rather than assuming the worst indefinitely.

The endpoint matters for a reason beyond nutrition. A diet with a planned end is psychologically different from an open ended restriction. It is a phase you are moving through, not a cage you are locked in, and that difference protects against the food anxiety that can outlast the physical condition entirely, a subject Chapter 12 takes up in full.

9.5 When Restriction Becomes the Problem

Sometimes the eating approach itself becomes the thing that needs treating, and it is worth seeing that clearly.

The following account is a composite, with details changed for anonymity.

Tatum had been managing methane overgrowth for two years, and over that time his diet had contracted to a very small number of foods he considered safe. Each new restriction had felt rational in the moment, added after a bad reaction. But the cumulative result was a diet so narrow that he had lost weight he could not afford to lose, dreaded eating anywhere outside his home, and had developed real anxiety around food. When he finally described his eating to a clinician, the restriction itself had become a more pressing problem than the overgrowth. The intervention was not another dietary rule. It was a careful, supported expansion of his diet, reintroducing foods methodically to show him how many he actually tolerated, alongside attention to the anxiety the long restriction had produced. His gut symptoms mattered, but they were no longer the only thing that needed care, and treating the overgrowth without addressing the shrunken, fearful eating would have solved half a problem while leaving the more disabling half in place.

Tatum's case is a warning about the direction restriction tends to drift if it is not bounded. What begins as a sensible tool becomes, without an endpoint and without attention, a condition of its own.

9.6 The Diet Is a Tool With an End

The eating approach for methane overgrowth is a balance, not a maximization. It lowers the fermentation that feeds your methane by reducing the most fermentable carbohydrates, while deliberately protecting the fiber and fluid your constipated gut needs to keep moving, and it does so as a bounded phase with a planned return to a wider diet, not as a permanent contraction (Villanueva-Millan et al., 2022). The governing principle throughout is the least restriction that works, because over restriction backfires in a constipated gut and corrodes your relationship with food.

Do this as you build your own approach. Instead of adding to a list of forbidden foods, start a short list of the specific foods that consistently, not occasionally, drive your symptoms, and treat that shorter list as your target rather than the sprawling one fear tends to generate. Set an endpoint for any restriction phase before you begin it, and plan the reintroduction that will follow. And hold onto the fact that the goal is a diet you can live in, not the narrowest one you can survive. The diet supports the treatment. It is not a punishment, and it is not the whole cure. With eating in its proper place, the book turns to the question that determines whether you will need to do any of this again, the search for why your gut became hospitable to overgrowth in the first place.

Chapter 10.0: Hunting the Root Cause

I just want to know why I have this. The clinician had heard the sentence a thousand times, but the patient in front of her said it with a particular exhaustion, the exhaustion of someone who had cleared her methane three times and relapsed three times and could not understand why her body kept regenerating the problem. She did not want another round of treatment. She wanted the reason. And she was right to want it, because until the reason is found, treatment is a bailing operation against a leak that never gets fixed. This chapter is about the hunt for that reason, the underlying driver that made your gut hospitable to overgrowth, because finding it is the difference between managing a condition forever and actually resolving it.

10.1 The Patient Who Wanted the Reason

The following account is a composite, with details changed for anonymity.

Tierney arrived having cleared her methane repeatedly and relapsed just as repeatedly, and she was done with treatment that did not last. She wanted to understand the cause. When her clinician took a genuinely thorough history rather than reaching for another prescription, several things surfaced that no previous treatment had considered. Tierney's constipation and slow transit had actually predated her overgrowth by years. She had been on a medication that reduces stomach acid for a long stretch. And there had been an episode, years earlier, of a severe gastrointestinal infection after travel, from which, in retrospect, her gut had never fully returned to normal.

None of these had been part of any prior treatment decision. Each had simply cleared her methane and sent her on her way, and each time the underlying conditions, the slow motility, the altered stomach acid, the possible aftermath of that infection, had sat there untouched, ready to let the overgrowth rebuild. The reframe changed everything about her care. Instead of asking how to clear the methane a fourth time, her clinician asked which of these drivers could be addressed so that clearing the methane might finally hold. The treatment that followed was not dramatically different in its antimicrobial phase, but it was aimed, for the first time, at the reasons the overgrowth kept returning rather than only at the overgrowth itself.

10.2 What Her Case Illustrates

Tierney's story illustrates the central concept of this chapter, which is that overgrowth is usually not a primary disease but a downstream consequence. Something makes the gut hospitable to overgrowth, and the overgrowth is the result. Treat the result without the cause, and the result returns.

This is why the earlier chapters kept insisting that clearing the organisms is only part of the job. The relapse rate, the self reinforcing loop, the centrality of motility, all of them point to the same underlying truth, that the overgrowth sits on top of some driver that treatment does not touch. The hunt for that driver is not an optional extra for the especially curious. It is the part of the process that determines whether you are heading toward resolution or toward a lifetime of re treatment.

The drivers are not exotic in most cases. They are a recognizable set of conditions and circumstances that impair the gut's defenses against overgrowth, and while identifying yours requires a clinician, understanding the categories lets you participate in the search rather than waiting passively for someone else to conduct it.

10.3 The Common Drivers

Several drivers account for most cases of overgrowth, and they are worth knowing by category.

The most important is impaired motility. The gut's between meal housekeeping wave, discussed in Chapter 8, is a primary defense against overgrowth, and anything that weakens it, a motility disorder, nerve or muscle problems affecting the gut, the aftermath of certain conditions, predisposes to accumulation of organisms (Ghoshal, 2011; Pimentel et al., 2020). For the methane patient, slow motility is doubly relevant, because it is both a common root cause and something the methane itself worsens.

A specific and well studied motility related driver is post infectious change. After an episode of gastroenteritis, food poisoning, a severe gut infection, some people develop lasting alterations in gut function, including impaired motility, that predispose to overgrowth and to the constellation often labeled irritable bowel syndrome (Pimentel et al., 2020). There is even antibody testing that can suggest a post infectious origin in some patients, which a gastroenterologist can discuss. Tierney's travel related infection, in retrospect, may have been exactly this kind of driver.

Other drivers include reduced stomach acid, whether from medications that suppress it or other causes, since stomach acid is part of the barrier that limits how many organisms reach and survive in the small intestine. Structural factors matter too, including the state of the valve between the small and large intestine, the aftermath of abdominal surgery, and adhesions or anatomical changes that impede normal flow. And various systemic conditions can impair gut motility or defenses as part of their broader effects. Which of these applies to you is a clinical question, but the categories give you a map of where to look.

10.4 The Framework for the Search

The practical framework is to treat root cause hunting as a structured conversation with a clinician rather than a guessing game.

It begins with a genuinely thorough history, the kind Tierney received, that asks when the symptoms truly began, what preceded them, what medications you take, what infections or surgeries you have had, and whether the constipation predated the overgrowth or followed it. That history often points toward the likely driver more efficiently than any test.

From there, specific investigations can be considered where the history warrants them, from the antibody testing that can suggest a post infectious origin to imaging or specialist assessment for suspected structural or motility problems (Pimentel et al., 2020). The point is not to run every possible test but to let the history direct a focused search. And where a driver is identified, the treatment plan can be aimed at it, addressing the reduced motility, adjusting a medication where appropriate and safe, managing an underlying condition, so that clearing the overgrowth has a chance to last.

This is also the juncture at which pushing for a gastroenterologist referral is most justified. Root cause work, particularly for suspected motility or structural drivers, often exceeds what primary care can investigate, and the next chapter takes up how to make that case effectively.

10.5 Two Searches, Two Outcomes

The value of the root cause hunt shows most clearly when you compare a search conducted with one skipped.

The following are composite cases.

Umber relapsed twice before a clinician took a full history and identified a longstanding motility problem as the likely driver of his repeated overgrowth. The plan that followed addressed the motility directly and sustainedly, not just the methane. His outcome was not a cure in the clean sense. He still needed attention to his gut and occasional adjustment. But the pattern of clearing and relapsing every few months resolved, because the driver underneath it was finally part of the treatment rather than an unexamined constant.

Vesper received excellent antimicrobial treatment three separate times, each course well chosen and effective at clearing her methane, and each time no one asked why her gut kept regenerating the problem. The root cause, whatever it was, was never sought. She relapsed after each course because the conditions that produced her overgrowth were never identified or addressed. Her treatment was not incompetent. It was incomplete, aimed repeatedly at the result and never once at the cause, and the result of that incompleteness was years of cycling that a serious root cause search might have shortened.

The contrast is not about the quality of the antimicrobial treatment, which was fine in both cases. It is about whether anyone looked underneath it. Umber's driver was found and addressed, and his cycling stopped. Vesper's was never sought, and her cycling continued. The difference between managing a condition indefinitely and moving toward resolution often comes down to exactly this, whether the hunt for the cause was conducted or skipped.

10.6 From Chasing to Finding

Your overgrowth is, in all likelihood, not a primary disease but a consequence of something that made your gut hospitable to it, most often impaired motility, sometimes a post infectious change, sometimes reduced stomach acid or a structural factor or a systemic condition (Ghoshal, 2011; Pimentel et al., 2020). Treatment aimed only at the overgrowth treats the consequence and leaves the cause in place, which is why so many patients clear their methane and relapse on a schedule. The hunt for the driver is what interrupts that pattern.

The implication for how you proceed is direct. Do not accept an endless series of re treatments without a serious search for why re treatment keeps being necessary. Bring your full history to a clinician, when the symptoms truly began, what preceded them, what you take, what you have been through, whether the constipation came before the overgrowth or after it, and press for that history to inform the search for a driver. Finding the cause does not always produce a perfect cure, but it changes the goal from chasing a recurring symptom to resolving the thing beneath it. That shift, from chasing to finding, is what turns treatment from a permanent condition of your life into a phase you can move through. The next chapter addresses the obstacle standing between many patients and all of this, the clinician who does not take the condition seriously in the first place.

Chapter 11.0: When Your Doctor Says IBS

Two patients walked into two appointments with the same complaint, chronic constipation and bloating, and the same suspicion, that something more specific than irritable bowel syndrome was going on. One walked out with a breath test requisition and a plan. The other walked out with a leaflet about fiber and the words it is just IBS still hanging in the air. The difference between them was not their bodies, which were remarkably similar, and it was not luck. It was almost entirely what they brought into the room and how they presented it. This chapter is about becoming the first patient, the one who is taken seriously, because for many people the hardest obstacle in this entire journey is not the biology of methane. It is getting a clinician to look past the reflexive label in the first place.

11.1 The Problem of the Reflexive Label

The problem is common and demoralizing. You describe symptoms that have upended your life, and they are folded, sometimes within a minute or two, into the diagnosis of irritable bowel syndrome, with the implication that little more can be done beyond fiber, fluid, and stress management. The word just often precedes IBS, as though the suffering were minor and the matter closed.

It helps to understand that this response is not always dismissiveness in the cruel sense. Irritable bowel syndrome is genuinely common, and it is a real diagnosis that fits many people. Some clinicians are also honestly skeptical of overgrowth as a concept, partly because the evidence base is uneven and partly because the topic has become surrounded by commercial noise and overselling of the kind this book keeps warning against. A degree of caution on their part is not entirely unreasonable. The trouble is that legitimate caution and reflexive dismissal look identical from the patient's chair, and both leave you without the specific investigation your symptoms may warrant.

The other half of the problem is access. Even a willing clinician may face limits on what testing is available, and even a correct suspicion of methane overgrowth may require a referral to a specialist who can investigate further. Getting past the reflexive label is therefore not only about persuasion. It is about presenting your case in a way that earns the next step, whether that is a test or a referral.

11.2 Why the Usual Approach Fails

Most patients approach the dismissive appointment in ways that, understandably, do not work.

One common approach is to arrive with a self diagnosis, announcing that you have methane SIBO or IMO and want it treated. This tends to raise a clinician's guard rather than lower it, because it can read as a patient who has decided the answer from the internet and wants the doctor to ratify it. Even when you are right, leading with the conclusion often triggers resistance.

Another common approach is to arrive with a diffuse, emotional recitation of years of suffering without structure. This is entirely human, and the suffering is real, but a clinician working within a short appointment struggles to convert an unstructured account into a specific next step. The very intensity of the distress can, unfairly, get folded into a mental health or stress framing rather than a gastrointestinal investigation.

A third approach is to accept the label quietly and leave, resolving to try harder with fiber, which is how many people spend years before finding a book like this one. The failure of these approaches is not a failure of the patient. It is a mismatch between how distress naturally presents and what a time pressured clinical encounter is built to act on.

11.3 The Pivot That Earns the Next Step

What changes the outcome is a shift from presenting suffering to presenting a case. The same facts, organized differently, move a clinician from reassurance toward investigation.

The pivot has a few elements. Instead of a self diagnosis, you bring specific, organized observations, the pattern of your symptoms, their timing, what has and has not helped, and crucially whether your constipation is the dominant feature. Instead of an unstructured recitation, you bring a concise summary a clinician can act on in the time available. And instead of asking for a particular treatment, you ask a specific, reasonable question, whether your constipation predominant, bloating heavy picture warrants a breath test for methane, given that methane on breath testing is consistently associated with constipation (Kunkel et al., 2011).

This works because it meets the clinician where they operate. You are not asking them to accept your diagnosis. You are giving them organized clinical information and asking a legitimate diagnostic question, which is exactly the kind of input a short appointment can convert into action. The North American Consensus and professional guidelines recognize breath testing for methane as a legitimate investigation in the right patient, so you are asking for something within the standard of care, not something fringe (Rezaie et al., 2017; Pimentel et al., 2020).

11.4 Two Appointments Compared

The difference the pivot makes is best seen directly.

The following are composite cases.

Fable prepared before her appointment. She brought a single page summarizing when her constipation began, its daily pattern, the bloating that worsened through the afternoon, the fiber and laxatives she had tried and their lack of effect, and a note that her dominant problem was constipation rather than diarrhea. She did not announce a diagnosis. She described the pattern and asked whether, given a constipation predominant picture, a breath test for methane might be worthwhile. Her clinician, presented with organized information and a specific reasonable question, agreed it was reasonable and arranged the test. The appointment took no longer than a dismissive one would have. What differed was what Fable brought into it.

Zephyr, with a nearly identical clinical picture, arrived without preparation and led by stating he was sure he had SIBO and wanted antibiotics. When the clinician hesitated, he became more insistent and then, running short on time, more distressed, describing years of suffering in an unstructured rush. The appointment ended with reassurance, a suggestion to increase fiber, and no test. Zephyr left convinced the clinician had not listened, which was partly true and partly a consequence of how the case had been presented. The same underlying condition that got Fable a test got Zephyr a leaflet.

The contrast is not about intelligence or deservingness. Both patients had the same condition and the same right to investigation. The difference was structure and framing, organized observations and a specific question versus a self diagnosis and an unstructured plea. That difference is learnable, which is the encouraging part.

11.5 Managing Expectations and Avoiding Harm

Preparing well does not guarantee an ideal response, and it is worth being realistic about the landscape you are entering.

Mainstream care and private or integrative care each offer something different, with different limits. Mainstream clinicians may be more cautious about overgrowth and more constrained in available testing, but they also operate within professional oversight and are less likely to sell you things. Private and integrative practitioners may be more willing to test and treat overgrowth, but the field contains a wide range of quality, and some patients have been both physically harmed and financially exploited by unregulated practitioners promoting aggressive and expensive regimens. Neither setting is uniformly better. Each requires a degree of informed vigilance.

Some warning signs are worth naming plainly. Be cautious of any practitioner who promises a definitive cure, who sells you large supplement packages directly from their own practice, who discourages you from involving a conventional physician, or who escalates treatment aggressively without clear reasoning. Confidence that outruns the evidence, which this book has flagged repeatedly as a feature of this space, is as much a warning sign in a practitioner as it is on a website. The same skepticism you would apply to a marketing claim applies to a person charging you for treatment.

The following account is a composite, with details changed for anonymity.

Fable, some months after finally getting her diagnosis, encountered the other side of the problem. Frustrated by slow progress, she consulted a practitioner who promised rapid, complete resolution and prescribed a long and costly list of supplements to be bought through his office, while suggesting she stop seeing her gastroenterologist. Something about the certainty unsettled her. She had learned, partly from the kind of honest framing this book tries to offer, that no one could reasonably promise a definitive cure for a condition whose evidence base is as uneven as this one's. She declined the package and stayed with her more measured, less dramatic conventional care. Her progress remained imperfect and gradual, which was, she came to understand, what honest treatment of this condition actually looks like. The practitioner's certainty had been the warning sign, not the reassurance it was dressed as.

11.6 The Case You Bring Them

Getting taken seriously is, to an uncomfortable degree, a skill separate from having a real condition, and the patients who get investigated are often simply the ones who present their case well. The obstacle is the reflexive label, sometimes dismissive and sometimes legitimately cautious, and the way past it is to shift from presenting suffering to presenting organized clinical information paired with a specific, reasonable question about testing for methane, which is a recognized investigation for the constipation predominant patient (Kunkel et al., 2011; Rezaie et al., 2017).

Prepare this before your next appointment. Write a single page with when your symptoms began, the daily pattern of your constipation and bloating, everything you have tried and its effect, and one clear line stating that constipation is your dominant problem. End it with the question you will ask, whether a breath test for methane is warranted given that picture. Bring it, hand a copy across if you can, and lead with the pattern rather than a diagnosis. If you are met with a flat refusal despite a reasonable case, it is legitimate to ask for a referral to a gastroenterologist, and to seek a second opinion. Choose any private practitioner with the same vigilance you would apply to any large purchase, and treat promises of a definitive cure as a reason to walk away rather than lean in. The case you build on that single page is the difference, more often than it should be, between another leaflet and an actual investigation. The final chapter turns inward, to the weight that carrying this condition places on you, and to why tending that weight is part of the treatment rather than separate from it.

Chapter 12.0: The Weight You Carry

Think about the ordinary act of deciding where to eat lunch. For most people it is a small pleasure or a passing logistical question. For someone who has lived with methane overgrowth for a while, that same small decision can carry a freight of calculation and dread, where is the bathroom, what can I safely order, will I be bloated and miserable by three o'clock, is it worth going at all. A condition that started in the gut has quietly migrated into the texture of daily life, into meals and plans and the willingness to leave the house. This chapter is about that migration, the mental and emotional weight of a chronic gut condition, and about why tending to it is not a soft addition to your treatment but a genuine part of it.

12.1 The Weight Is Real and It Is Physical Too

The central idea of this chapter is that the burden of this condition is not confined to your intestines, and that the mind and the gut are connected in ways that make the emotional weight a legitimate clinical concern rather than a distraction from the real problem.

The connection runs in both directions. Chronic gut symptoms produce real psychological strain, anxiety about symptoms and food and access to bathrooms, low mood from the grind of a condition that will not resolve, exhaustion from years of trying. And that psychological strain in turn affects the gut, because the gut and the nervous system are in constant communication, and stress and anxiety measurably influence gut function, including motility, the very thing your condition already compromises (Pimentel et al., 2020). This is not a matter of the symptoms being in your head. It is a matter of a genuine two way relationship in which distress and gut dysfunction feed each other.

This bidirectional link is why the emotional weight cannot be dismissed as separate from the physical condition. Anxiety that worsens motility worsens the exact mechanism driving your constipation. Attending to the weight is therefore not a departure from treating the gut. In a real sense it is part of it.

12.2 How the Weight Accumulates

The weight rarely arrives all at once. It accumulates, one reasonable adaptation at a time, until it has reshaped a life.

It often begins with food. After enough bad reactions, eating starts to feel dangerous, and the list of safe foods contracts, a process Chapter 9 examined from the dietary side. From the psychological side, this is the growth of food anxiety, a state in which meals become a source of fear rather than nourishment or pleasure. The restriction that began as a treatment tool becomes a cage, and the fear can outlast the physical symptoms that started it.

It spreads to activity and social life. The unpredictability of the gut makes leaving home feel risky, and people begin declining invitations, avoiding restaurants, planning their days around bathroom access. The world shrinks. Isolation grows, and with it the low mood that isolation breeds.

And it settles into identity. After enough years and enough failed treatments, some people come to see themselves as fundamentally broken, as someone whose body does not work, and that self perception colors everything. This is where the grind becomes genuinely heavy, when a gut condition has become a story a person tells about their whole self.

Naming this accumulation matters, because each step felt reasonable in isolation and only the sum reveals how much has been given up. Seeing the pattern is the first step toward interrupting it.

12.3 What Actually Helps

Several things help with the weight, and none of them are platitudes.

The first is accurate understanding, which is much of what this book has tried to provide. A great deal of the anxiety around this condition comes from confusion and from the sense of an unpredictable, inexplicable body. Understanding the mechanism, why the constipation happens, why treatment sometimes fails, what actually helps, replaces mystery with something a person can reason about, and that shift alone reduces the fear considerably. Knowledge is not merely practical here. It is calming.

The second is realistic expectations. Much of the despair in this condition comes from expecting a clean cure and experiencing each relapse as a catastrophic failure. This book has been honest that improvement is often gradual and partial, that relapse is common and does not mean the treatment failed, and that the realistic goal is usually good management rather than perfect resolution. Holding that expectation changes how setbacks feel. A relapse understood as an expected part of a manageable condition is a very different experience from a relapse understood as proof that nothing works.

The third is attending to the anxiety directly, rather than waiting for the gut symptoms to resolve first. Because the relationship between distress and gut function runs both ways, managing anxiety and low mood can support gut function even as the physical treatment proceeds (Pimentel et al., 2020). Stress management is not a consolation prize offered when medicine has nothing else. It is a lever on the same system.

The fourth, and it deserves to be said plainly, is professional support when the weight becomes heavy enough. Persistent anxiety, low mood that does not lift, food fear that is narrowing your life, or a sense of hopelessness that colors your days are all reasons to seek help from a mental health professional, and doing so is not an admission that the condition is imaginary. It is appropriate care for a real burden. If the weight of this has become hard to carry, talking to your doctor or a mental health professional about that part, specifically, is a reasonable and worthwhile step.

12.4 Two Ways of Carrying It

The difference that tending to the weight makes shows in how two people carry the same condition.

The following are composite cases.

Yael had methane overgrowth and, alongside her physical treatment, took the emotional side seriously. She learned the mechanism of her condition, which reduced the fear that had surrounded it. She held realistic expectations, so that a relapse felt like an expected bump rather than a collapse. And when her food anxiety began narrowing her life, she sought support for it directly rather than waiting for her gut to be perfect first. Her physical condition improved gradually and imperfectly, much like anyone's. But she carried it differently, as a manageable part of her life rather than the defining fact of it, and that difference was not cosmetic. Her reduced anxiety supported the very motility her treatment was working on.

Zennor had a similar physical condition and comparable physical treatment, but the weight went unattended. Each relapse landed as a catastrophe because he expected a cure. His food anxiety grew unchecked until his diet and his social life had both contracted sharply. He came to see himself as broken, and that self perception deepened the low mood and the isolation, which in turn, through the two way link between distress and the gut, gave his symptoms one more thing to feed on. His physical treatment was reasonable. What was missing was any attention to the accumulating weight, and its absence made everything harder, including the physical condition itself.

The two men had the same illness and carried it toward different lives. The difference was not the severity of the overgrowth. It was whether the weight was acknowledged and tended or left to accumulate unexamined.

12.5 A Word Against a Common Story

There is a particular story this condition tempts people to tell, and it is worth arguing against directly, because it does real harm.

The story is that a body which has failed to respond to treatment, which stays constipated and bloated despite every effort, is a broken body, and that the person inhabiting it is somehow at fault, insufficiently disciplined or simply defective. This story is false on the evidence. Your condition, as this entire book has laid out, has understandable mechanisms and identifiable drivers, and treatment failures are usually mismatches or incomplete approaches rather than verdicts on you (Pimentel et al., 2020; Low et al., 2010). The gut that keeps regenerating overgrowth is not a moral failing. It is a system with a driver that has not yet been found or fully addressed.

Replacing that story matters not only because it is kinder but because it is more accurate, and because the harsh version actively worsens things. Self blame feeds the anxiety and low mood that, through the gut brain link, feed the symptoms. The accurate story, that this is a mechanistic condition you are working to manage, not a punishment you are failing to escape, is both truer and more useful.

12.6 The Weight You Can Set Down

The burden of methane overgrowth extends well beyond the gut, into food and plans and self perception, and it is connected to the physical condition through a genuine two way relationship in which distress and gut dysfunction feed each other (Pimentel et al., 2020). This is why the emotional weight is not a separate matter to be handled once the real problem is solved. It is part of the real problem, and tending to it supports the physical treatment rather than distracting from it.

The reframe to carry out of this book is that some of this weight can be set down, and setting it down is legitimate treatment, not indulgence. Accurate understanding replaces fear with reasoning. Realistic expectations turn relapse from catastrophe into an expected part of a manageable condition. Attending to anxiety supports the very motility your treatment targets. And seeking professional help when the weight grows heavy is appropriate care, not surrender. You did not fail your way into this condition, and you will not discipline your way out of it. You will manage it, gradually and imperfectly and with the whole of yourself accounted for, gut and mind together, because they were never really separate. That is not a smaller ambition than a cure. For a condition like this one, it is the realistic shape of actually getting your life back.

Conclusion: Your Methane Specific Plan

Everything in this book unfolds from a single correction. What you have been calling bacterial overgrowth is very likely archaeal, driven by methanogens that make methane, and that one fact reorganizes the entire picture. It explains why you are constipated rather than loose, because methane slows the gut. It explains why the standard single antibiotic disappointed you, because that drug was built for bacteria and your organisms belong to a separate branch of life. It explains why your treatment keeps unraveling, because clearing the organisms without repairing the sluggish motility that let them accumulate leaves the loop intact. And it explains why the reclassification to intestinal methanogen overgrowth is more than a new acronym. The name carries the mechanism, and the mechanism points at what helps.

The plan that follows from all of this is not a single act but a sequence, and it is worth holding the whole of it in view. It begins with reading your own breath test accurately, applying the methane threshold correctly, and judging the result against your lived symptoms. It moves to treatment aimed at archaea rather than bacteria, most often a combined antimicrobial approach for methane, understood well enough to discuss with a prescriber and never attempted alone. It considers herbal options honestly, as a plausible but less established alternative rather than a guaranteed cure. It places motility support at the center, because the maintenance phase, not the antimicrobial phase, is where durable change lives. It uses diet as a bounded tool, lowering fermentation without starving the constipated gut, with a planned return to a wider way of eating. It hunts for the root cause, the driver underneath the overgrowth, so that clearing the methane has a chance to last. It equips you to get taken seriously by a clinician in the first place. And it accounts for the weight the condition places on the rest of your life, because the gut and the mind are not separable and tending one supports the other.

None of this promises a clean cure, and this book has refused to pretend otherwise, because the honest evidence does not support that promise and because you have almost certainly been burned by promises that did. What it offers instead is understanding and leverage. You now know what your condition actually is, why it behaves as it does, and what genuinely helps, graded honestly by how strong the evidence behind it is. That knowledge turns you from a patient waiting to be handed a leaflet into one who can hold a real conversation with the clinician able to help, ask the right questions, recognize the wrong answers, and participate in the decisions about your own body.

Do one last thing before you close the book. On a single page, write your plan as it stands today. Note your highest methane reading and whether it fit your symptoms. Note the treatment approach you intend to discuss with a prescriber, combined antimicrobial or supervised herbal, and the questions you will ask about it. Note your motility plan, including meal spacing and any prokinetic to raise with your clinician. Note the dietary boundaries you are choosing and the endpoint you have set for any restriction. Note the root cause worth investigating given your history. And note a review date, a point at which you will take stock rather than drifting. That single page is the distilled use of everything here, and it is yours to carry into the rooms where the actual decisions get made. The overgrowth was never ordinary, and now, neither is your understanding of it.

Appendix A: IMO Compared With the Other Subtypes

Intestinal methanogen overgrowth is one of several gas defined patterns, and seeing them side by side clarifies where yours sits. Hydrogen dominant overgrowth involves ordinary bacteria producing hydrogen, tends toward diarrhea or looser stools and urgency, and often responds to a single nonabsorbable antibiotic. Methane dominant overgrowth, the subject of this book, involves methanogenic archaea producing methane, tends strongly toward constipation and trapped bloating, and responds better to a combined antimicrobial approach paired with motility support than to a single drug. A third pattern, associated with hydrogen sulfide, has its own features and is measured on newer tests. The organizing insight is that the gas defines the subtype, the subtype predicts the dominant symptom, and the subtype should shape the treatment. Filing all of these under one label obscures exactly the distinctions that determine what will help you.

Appendix B: Your Appointment Summary Sheet

Bring a single page to your appointment containing the following. When your symptoms first began, and what, if anything, preceded them. The daily pattern of your constipation, including how many days you typically go between bowel movements. The pattern of your bloating, including when in the day it worsens. Everything you have tried, fiber, laxatives, diets, prior antibiotics, and what effect each had. One clear sentence stating that constipation is your dominant problem, if it is. Any breath test results you have, with the highest methane value and its time point. And the question you intend to ask, whether a breath test for methane is warranted given a constipation predominant picture, or, if already diagnosed, whether a combined approach and a motility plan are appropriate. Hand a copy across if you can. Organized information plus a specific question is what converts a short appointment into a next step.

Appendix C: Symptom and Transit Tracker

A simple tracker, kept over several weeks, gives you and your clinician far better information than memory alone. Each day, note whether you had a bowel movement and its general character, the timing and severity of any bloating, what you ate in broad terms, the gaps between your meals and the length of your overnight fast, and any medications or supplements taken. Over time, patterns emerge that are invisible day to day, which foods consistently rather than occasionally drive symptoms, whether longer meal gaps ease the bloating, whether a treatment is holding or fading. Bring the tracker to appointments. It turns vague impressions into evidence.

Appendix D: The Evidence Confidence Key

Throughout this book, claims have been graded honestly, and it helps to know what the grades mean. Some claims rest on strong physiology and repeated observation, such as the fact that methane slows intestinal transit, and these can be relied on with reasonable confidence. Some rest on smaller studies or retrospective reviews, such as the specific eradication figures for combined antimicrobial therapy, and these are well supported but should not be treated as precise or guaranteed. Some rest on limited evidence, such as the effectiveness of herbal protocols specifically for methane, and these are plausible but genuinely uncertain. The professional guidelines themselves rate much of the overgrowth evidence base as low or very low quality. Knowing which grade a claim carries is what lets you weigh it properly and recognize overselling when you meet it.

Appendix E: Questions Worth Asking

For a prescriber considering treatment, ask whether your methane result supports a combined approach rather than a single drug, what second agent would be used and why, what its trade offs are for you specifically, and how the plan addresses motility and relapse rather than only the immediate overgrowth. For any practitioner, conventional or integrative, be wary if they promise a definitive cure, sell you large supplement packages directly, discourage you from involving a conventional physician, or escalate treatment aggressively without clear reasoning. Confidence that outruns the evidence is a warning sign in a person as much as on a website.

Appendix F: A Short Glossary

Archaea, a separate domain of life from bacteria, including the methanogens that cause this condition. Methanogen, an archaeon that produces methane, chiefly the species that overgrows in your gut. Intestinal methanogen overgrowth, the current name for methane dominant overgrowth, reflecting that the culprits are methanogens and that they range beyond the small intestine. Cross feeding, the relationship in which bacteria produce hydrogen that methanogens consume to make methane. Migrating motor complex, the between meal housekeeping wave that sweeps the small intestine and defends against overgrowth. Prokinetic, an agent that supports gut motility, used to help prevent relapse. Parts per million, the unit in which breath test gases are measured, with a methane reading of ten or more at any point defining overgrowth.

Appendix G: A Note on Sources and Further Reading

The claims in this book are drawn from peer reviewed research, professional guidelines, and consensus statements, listed in full in the references that follow. The most useful anchors for a reader who wishes to go further are the North American Consensus on breath testing and the American College of Gastroenterology clinical guideline on overgrowth, both of which lay out the diagnostic thresholds and treatment logic in professional terms, and the primary studies on methane and transit, on combined antimicrobial treatment, and on relapse prevention through motility support. When reading further, apply the same standard this book has tried to model. Prefer primary research and professional guidelines over commercial content, and treat confident promises of a cure with the skepticism the uneven evidence base warrants.

References

Chedid, V., Dhalla, S., Clarke, J. O., Roland, B. C., Dunbar, K. B., Koh, J., Justino, E., Tomakin, E., & Mullin, G. E. (2014). Herbal therapy is equivalent to rifaximin for the treatment of small intestinal bacterial overgrowth. Global Advances in Health and Medicine, 3(3), 16-24. https://doi.org/10.7453/gahmj.2014.019

Ghoshal, U. C. (2011). How to interpret hydrogen breath tests. Journal of Neurogastroenterology and Motility, 17(3), 312-317. https://doi.org/10.5056/jnm.2011.17.3.312

Kunkel, D., Basseri, R. J., Makhani, M. D., Chong, K., Chang, C., & Pimentel, M. (2011). Methane on breath testing is associated with constipation: A systematic review and meta-analysis. Digestive Diseases and Sciences, 56(6), 1612-1618. https://doi.org/10.1007/s10620-011-1590-5

Low, K., Hwang, L., Hua, J., Zhu, A., Morales, W., & Pimentel, M. (2010). A combination of rifaximin and neomycin is most effective in treating irritable bowel syndrome patients with methane on lactulose breath test. Journal of Clinical Gastroenterology, 44(8), 547-550. https://doi.org/10.1097/MCG.0b013e3181c64c90

Pimentel, M., Soffer, E. E., Chow, E. J., Kong, Y., & Lin, H. C. (2002). Lower frequency of MMC is found in IBS subjects with abnormal lactulose breath test, suggesting bacterial overgrowth. Digestive Diseases and Sciences, 47(12), 2639-2643. https://doi.org/10.1023/A:1021039032413

Pimentel, M., Lin, H. C., Enayati, P., van den Burg, B., Lee, H. R., Chen, J. H., Park, S., Kong, Y., & Conklin, J. (2006a). Methane, a gas produced by enteric bacteria, slows intestinal transit and augments small intestinal contractile activity.

American Journal of Physiology Gastrointestinal and Liver Physiology, 290(6), G1089-G1095. https://doi.org/10.1152/ajpgi.00574.2004

Pimentel, M., Chatterjee, S., Chow, E. J., Park, S., & Kong, Y. (2006b). Neomycin improves constipation-predominant irritable bowel syndrome in a fashion that is dependent on the presence of methane gas: Subanalysis of a double-blind randomized controlled study. Digestive Diseases and Sciences, 51(8), 1297-1301. https://doi.org/10.1007/s10620-006-9104-6

Pimentel, M., Morales, W., Lezcano, S., Sun-Chuan, D., Low, K., & Yang, J. (2009). Low-dose nocturnal tegaserod or erythromycin delays symptom recurrence after treatment of irritable bowel syndrome based on presumed bacterial overgrowth. Gastroenterology and Hepatology, 5(6), 435-442.

Pimentel, M., Saad, R. J., Long, M. D., & Rao, S. S. C. (2020). ACG clinical guideline: Small intestinal bacterial overgrowth. American Journal of Gastroenterology, 115(2), 165-178. https://doi.org/10.14309/ajg.0000000000000501

Rezaie, A., Buresi, M., Lembo, A., Lin, H., McCallum, R., Rao, S., Schmulson, M., Valdovinos, M., Zakko, S., & Pimentel, M. (2017). Hydrogen and methane-based breath testing in gastrointestinal disorders: The North American Consensus. American Journal of Gastroenterology, 112(5), 775-784. https://doi.org/10.1038/ajg.2017.46

Saad, R. J., & Chey, W. D. (2014). Breath testing for small intestinal bacterial overgrowth: Maximizing test accuracy. Clinical Gastroenterology and Hepatology, 12(12), 1964-1972. https://doi.org/10.1016/j.cgh.2013.09.055

Shah, S. C., Day, L. W., Somsouk, M., & Sewell, J. L. (2013). Meta-analysis: Antibiotic therapy for small intestinal bacterial overgrowth. Alimentary Pharmacology and Therapeutics, 38(8), 925-934. https://doi.org/10.1111/apt.12479

Suri, J., Kataria, R., Malik, Z., Parkman, H. P., & Schey, R. (2018). Elevated methane levels in small intestinal bacterial overgrowth suggests delayed small bowel and colonic transit. Medicine (Baltimore), 97(21), e10554. https://doi.org/10.1097/MD.0000000000010554

Takakura, W., Pimentel, M., Rao, S., Villanueva-Millan, M. J., Chang, C., Morales, W., Sanchez, M., Torosyan, J., Rashid, M., Hosseini, A., Wang, J., Leite, G., Kowalewski, E., Mathur, R., & Rezaie, A. (2022). A single fasting exhaled methane level correlates with fecal methanogen load, clinical symptoms and accurately detects intestinal methanogen overgrowth. American Journal of Gastroenterology, 117(3), 470-477. https://doi.org/10.14309/ajg.0000000000001607

Villanueva-Millan, M. J., Leite, G., Wang, J., Morales, W., Parodi, G., Pimentel, M. L., Barlow, G. M., Mathur, R., Rezaie, A., Sanchez, M., Ayyad, S., Cohrs, D., Chang, C., Rashid, M., Hosseini, A., Fiorentino, A., Weitsman, S., Chuang, B., Chang, B., . . . Pimentel, M. (2022). Methanogens and hydrogen sulfide producing bacteria guide distinct gut microbe profiles and irritable bowel syndrome subtypes. American Journal of Gastroenterology, 117(12), 2055-2066. https://doi.org/10.14309/ajg.0000000000001997

www.ingramcontent.com/pod-product-compliance
Lightning Source LLC
LaVergne TN
LVHW022307200926
848481LV00004B/1239
9798905992964